Problem Solving in Pa

Inte

You treat a disease, you win, you lose. You treat a person, I guarantee you, you'll win, no matter what the outcome.

Hunter Doherty 'Patch' Adams, MD (American physician, author and social activist)

Problem Solving
in Patient-Centred and
Integrated Cancer Care

Edited by

Galina Velikova, BMBS, PhD, FRCP
Professor of Psychosocial and Medical Oncology, Leeds Institute of Cancer and
Pathology, University of Leeds, Leeds; Leeds Cancer Centre, St James's University Hospital,
Leeds Teaching Hospitals NHS Trust, Leeds

Lesley Fallowfield, DBE, BSc, DPhil, FMedSci
Director, Sussex Health Outcomes Research and Education in Cancer (SHORE-C),
University of Sussex, Brighton

Jane Younger, MBChB, MRCPsych
Consultant in Psychological Medicine, Clatterbridge Cancer Centre NHS Foundation
Trust, Birkenhead

Ruth E. Board, BSc, MBChB, PhD, FRCP
Consultant in Medical Oncology, Lancashire Teaching Hospitals NHS Foundation Trust,
Preston; Honorary Senior Lecturer, University of Manchester, Manchester

Peter Selby, CBE, MD, MA, DSc, FRCP, FRCR, FMedSci
Professor of Cancer Medicine and Associate Dean, University of Leeds and Leeds
Teaching Hospitals NHS Trust, Leeds; Honorary President of the Association of Cancer
Physicians and of the European Cancer Concord

Published in association with the Association of Cancer Physicians

EBN HEALTH

OXFORD, UK

EBN Health
An imprint of Evidence-based Networks Ltd
Witney Business & Innovation Centre
Windrush House, Burford Road
Witney, Oxfordshire OX29 7DX, UK

Tel: +44 1865 522326
Email: info@ebnhealth.com

Web: www.ebnhealth.com

Distributed worldwide by:
Marston Book Services Ltd
160 Eastern Avenue
Milton Park
Abingdon
Oxon OX14 4SB, UK
Tel: +44 1235 465500
Fax: +44 1235 465555
Email: trade.orders@marston.co.uk

Although every effort has been made to ensure that all owners of copyright material have been acknowledged in this publication, we would be glad to acknowledge in subsequent reprints or editions any omissions brought to the attention in writing of EBN Health or Evidence-based Networks Ltd.

EBN Health and Evidence-based Networks Ltd bear no responsibility for the persistence or accuracy of URLs for external or third-party internet websites referred to in this publication, and do not guarantee that any content on such websites is, or will remain, accurate or appropriate.

A catalogue record for this book is available from the British Library.

ISBN 13   978 0 99559 540 8
ISBN e-book 978 0 99559 541 5

The publisher makes no representation, express or implied, that the dosages in this book are correct. Readers must therefore always check the product information and clinical procedures with the most up-to-date published product information and data sheets provided by the manufacturers and the most recent codes of conduct and safety regulations. The authors and the publisher do not accept any liability for any errors in the text or for the misuse or misapplication of material in this work.

Series design by Pete Russell Typographic Design, Faringdon, Oxon, UK
Typeset by Ian Winter Design, Ramsden, Oxon, UK
Printed by Latimer Trend and Company Ltd, Plymouth, UK

Contents

Contributors

Dr Helen Adderley, Registrar in Medical Oncology, Christie NHS Foundation Trust, Manchester

Assistant Professor Tit Albreht, Senior Health Services Researcher, Head of Centre for Health Care, National Institute of Public Health of Slovenia, Ljubljana, Slovenia

Dr Anne Armstrong, Consultant in Medical Oncology and Honorary Senior Lecturer, Christie NHS Foundation Trust, Manchester

Professor Michael I. Bennett, St Gemma's Professor of Palliative Medicine, Leeds Institute of Health Sciences, University of Leeds, Leeds

Dr Christine Berling, Head of International and European Affairs, Directorate General for Health, Ministry of Health and Solidarity, Paris, France

Dr Ruth E. Board, Consultant in Medical Oncology, Lancashire Teaching Hospitals NHS Foundation Trust, Preston; Honorary Senior Lecturer, University of Manchester, Manchester

Mr Hugh Butcher, Cancer Patient Advocate and University of Leeds Visiting Research Fellow (Patient and Public Involvement), Leeds Institute of Cancer and Pathology, University of Leeds, Leeds

Dr Josie Butcher, Consultant and Director, Psychosexual Medicine and Therapy Service, Cheshire and Wirral Partnership NHS Foundation Trust, Chester

Dr Lynn Calman, Senior Research Fellow, Macmillan Survivorship Research Group, Faculty of Health Sciences, University of Southampton, Southampton

Dr Kate Cardale, Consultant in Clinical Oncology, Leeds Cancer Centre, St James's University Hospital, Leeds Teaching Hospitals NHS Trust, Leeds

Mrs Anne Carter, Advanced Oncology Team Leader Dietitian, Lancashire Teaching Hospitals NHS Foundation Trust, Preston

Dr Meera Chauhan, Clinical Research Fellow, University of Leicester, Leicester

Dr Vinton Cheng, Clinical Research Fellow, CRUK/MRC Oxford Institute for Radiation Oncology, Department of Oncology, University of Oxford, Oxford

Dr Sinead Clarke, GP Adviser, Macmillan Cancer Support, London

Miss Kate Cleary, Administrative Officer, Wales Cancer Research Centre, Cardiff University, Cardiff

Dr Laura Clipsham, Consultant in Palliative Medicine, Leicester Royal Infirmary, University Hospitals of Leicester NHS Trust, Leicester

Mrs Tracey Coleby, Macmillan Breast Palliative Care Clinical Nurse Specialist, Christie NHS Foundation Trust, Manchester

Dr Alicia-Marie Conway, Specialist Registrar in Medical Oncology, Christie NHS Foundation Trust, Manchester

Dr Anthony Cunliffe, Macmillan Lead GP Adviser for Prevention and Diagnosis, Macmillan Cancer Support, London

Dr Iva Damyanova, Consultant in Medical Oncology, Mid-Yorkshire Hospitals NHS Trust, Wakefield

Ms Bethan Daniel, Macmillan Secondary Breast Clinical Nurse Specialist, Christie NHS Foundation Trust, Manchester

Dr Gemma Dart, Registrar in Medical Oncology, Leeds Cancer Centre, St James's University Hospital, Leeds Teaching Hospitals NHS Trust, Leeds

Professor Sean Duffy, West Yorkshire and Harrogate Cancer Alliance Lead, Leeds

Dr Ladislav Dusek, Head of Department, Institute for Biostatistics and Analyses, Faculty of Medicine, Masaryk University, Czechia

Mrs Katy Everson, Specialist Dietitian in Oncology, Royal Preston Hospital, Lancashire Teaching Hospitals NHS Foundation Trust, Preston

Professor Dame Lesley Fallowfield, Director, Sussex Health Outcomes Research and Education in Cancer (SHORE-C), University of Sussex, Brighton

Dr Claudia Ferrari, Head of Department of Care Organization, French National Cancer Institute (INCa), Boulogne Billancourt, France

Mr Andrew Fishburn, Lead Clinical Nurse Specialist in Head and Neck, Lancashire Teaching Hospitals NHS Foundation Trust, Preston

Dr Jim Fitzgibbon, Volunteer Lead Research Partner, Wales Cancer Research Centre, Cardiff University, Cardiff

Dr Lucy Flanders, Core Medical Trainee, National Medical Director's Clinical Fellow, NHS England, London

Dr Nicola Flaum, Specialist Registrar in Medical Oncology, Christie NHS Foundation Trust, Manchester

Professor Claire Foster, Professor of Psychosocial Oncology and Director of Macmillan Survivorship Research Group, Faculty of Health Sciences, University of Southampton, Southampton

Dr Alexandra Gilbert, NIHR Academic Clinical Lecturer in Clinical Oncology, University of Leeds; Leeds Cancer Centre, St James's University Hospital, Leeds Teaching Hospitals NHS Trust, Leeds

Dr Justin Grayer, Principal Clinical Psychologist and Psychosexual and Relationship Therapist, Lead of Adult Psychological Support Team, Royal Marsden NHS Foundation Trust, London

Dr Geoff Hall, Senior Lecturer in Medical Oncology, Leeds Institute of Cancer and Pathology, University of Leeds, Leeds; Leeds Cancer Centre, St James's University Hospital, Leeds Teaching Hospitals NHS Trust, Leeds

Dr Jurjees Hasan, Consultant in Medical Oncology, Christie NHS Foundation Trust, Manchester

Miss Rachel Hewitson, Macmillan Speech and Language Therapist, Lancashire Teaching Hospitals NHS Foundation Trust, Preston

Dr Nicola Hughes, Academic Clinical Fellow in Medical Oncology, Leeds Cancer Centre, St James's University Hospital, Leeds Teaching Hospitals NHS Trust, Leeds

Dr Fiona James, Foundation Doctor, Royal Preston Hospital, Lancashire Teaching Hospitals NHS Foundation Trust, Preston

Professor Stein Kaasa, Head of Department of Oncology, Oslo University Hospital and University of Oslo, Oslo, Norway

Dr Suryanarayana Kakkilaya, Consultant in Psychiatry, Elysium Healthcare, Warrington

Dr Clare Kane, Registrar in Clinical Oncology, North Middlesex University Hospital NHS Trust, London

Dr Sam Khan, Clinical Research Fellow, University of Leicester, Leicester

Dr Hariharan Kuhan, Specialist Registrar in Medical Oncology, Mount Vernon Cancer Centre, Northwood, Middlesex

Ms Laura Lee, CEO, Maggie's Centres, London

Dr Rebecca Lee, Specialist Registrar, Christie NHS Foundation Trust, Manchester

Dr Pauline Leonard, Consultant in Medical Oncology, Whittington Health NHS Trust, London

Dr Alexandra R. Lewis, Specialist Registrar in Medical Oncology, Christie NHS Foundation Trust, Manchester

Dr Kok Haw Jonathan Lim, Specialty Trainee in Medical Oncology, Christie NHS Foundation Trust, Manchester

Dr Oana C. Lindner, Research Fellow, Patient-Centred Outcomes Research Group, University of Leeds, Leeds

Dr Kim Linton, Consultant in Medical Oncology, Christie NHS Foundation Trust, Manchester

Dr Fotios Loupakis, Consultant in Medical Oncology, Azienda University Hospital, Pisa, Italy

Dr Emma Lowe, Consultant in Palliative Medicine, Mid Yorkshire Hospitals NHS Trust, Wakefield

Professor Lucio Luzzatto, Honorary Professor of Haematology, University of Florence, Florence, Italy

Dr Jane Maher, Joint Chief Medical Officer, Macmillan Cancer Support, London; Honorary Consultant in Clinical Oncology, Mount Vernon Cancer Centre, Northwood, Middlesex

Dr Lucinda Melcher, Consultant in Clinical Oncology, North Middlesex University Hospital NHS Trust, London

Dr Maung Maung Myat Moe, Consultant in Medical Oncology, North Middlesex University Hospital NHS Trust, London

Dr Mulyati Mohamed, Specialty Doctor in Medical Oncology, Whittington Health NHS Trust, London

Dr Siobhan Morrison, Registrar in Clinical Oncology, Christie NHS Foundation Trust, Manchester

Dr Paul Nathan, Consultant in Medical Oncology, Mount Vernon Cancer Centre, Northwood, Middlesex

Professor Richard D. Neal, Professor of Primary Care Oncology, University of Leeds, Leeds

Dr Annmarie Nelson, Scientific Director, Marie Curie Research Centre, Cardiff University, Cardiff

Dr Pete Nightingale, GP Adviser End of Life Care, Macmillan Cancer Support, Lancaster

Dr Anna Olsson-Brown, Registrar in Medical Oncology, Clatterbridge Cancer Centre NHS Foundation Trust, Birkenhead; Clinical Research Fellow, University of Liverpool, Liverpool

Dr Mark Openshaw, Clinical Research Fellow, University of Leicester, Leicester

Dr Louisa Petchey, Senior Policy Analyst, Macmillan Cancer Support, London

Ms Gail Prout, Skin Cancer Clinical Nurse Specialist, Mount Vernon Cancer Centre, Northwood, Middlesex

Dr Dulani Ranatunge, Specialist Registrar in Medical Oncology, Leeds Cancer Centre, St James's University Hospital, Leeds Teaching Hospitals NHS Trust, Leeds

Dr Charlotte Richardson, Registrar in Medical Oncology, Leeds Cancer Centre, St James's University Hospital, Leeds Teaching Hospitals NHS Trust, Leeds

Dr Lesley Seddon, Consultant in Health Psychology (Oncology) and Head of Psychology Services, Royal Preston Hospital, Lancashire Teaching Hospitals NHS Foundation Trust, Preston

Professor Peter Selby, Professor of Cancer Medicine and Associate Dean, Leeds Institute of Cancer and Pathology, University of Leeds, Leeds; Leeds Cancer Centre, St James's University Hospital, Leeds Teaching Hospitals NHS Trust, Leeds

Dr Richard Simcock, Consultant in Clinical Oncology, Sussex Cancer Centre, Brighton and Sussex University Hospitals NHS Trust, Brighton

Mrs Cate Simmons, Upper GI and CUP Clinical Nurse Specialist, Princess Alexandra Hospital, Harlow

Dr Muthiah Sivaramalingam, Consultant in Clinical Oncology, Royal Preston Hospital, Lancashire Teaching Hospitals NHS Foundation Trust, Preston

Dr Lesley Smith, Consequences of Treatment Programme Manager, Macmillan Cancer Support, London

Dr Dan Stark, Consultant in Medical Oncology, Leeds Cancer Centre, St James's University Hospital, Leeds Teaching Hospitals NHS Trust, Leeds

Dr Jacqui Stringer, Clinical Lead, Tissue Viability and Complementary Health and Wellbeing, Christie NHS Foundation Trust, Manchester; Honorary Lecturer, University of Manchester, Manchester

Dr Daniel Swinson, Consultant in Medical Oncology, Leeds Cancer Centre, St James's University Hospital, Leeds Teaching Hospitals NHS Trust, Leeds

Dr Elena Takeuchi, Consultant in Medical Oncology, Christie NHS Foundation Trust, Manchester

Professor Denis Talbot, Professor of Cancer Medicine, Churchill Hospital, Oxford University Hospitals NHS Foundation Trust, Oxford

Professor Anne Thomas, Professor of Cancer Therapeutics, University of Leicester, Leicester

Dr Luzia Travado, Head of Psycho-Oncology, Champalimaud Clinical Centre, Champalimaud Foundation, Lisbon, Portugal

Miss Lorraine Turner, Advanced Nurse Practitioner in Experimental Cancer Medicine, NIHR/Cancer Research UK Christie Clinical Research Facility, Christie NHS Foundation Trust, Manchester

Dr Rob Turner, Operational Lead Cancer Clinician, Leeds Cancer Centre, Leeds Teaching Hospitals NHS Trust, Leeds

Professor Galina Velikova, Professor of Psychosocial and Medical Oncology, Leeds Institute of Cancer and Pathology, University of Leeds, Leeds; Leeds Cancer Centre, St James's University Hospital, Leeds Teaching Hospitals NHS Trust, Leeds

Mr Pete Wallroth, CEO/Founder, Mummy's Star charity (www.mummysstar.org)

Professor Andrew M. Wardley, Medical Director, NIHR Cancer Research UK Christie Clinical Research Facility, Christie NHS Foundation Trust, Manchester; Division of Cancer Sciences, University of Manchester, Manchester

Dr Isabel White, Clinical Research Fellow in Psychosexual Practice, Royal Marsden NHS Foundation Trust, London

Dr Penny Wright, Associate Professor in Psychosocial Cancer Care, Leeds Institute of Cancer and Pathology, University of Leeds, Leeds

Dr Alison Young, Consultant in Medical Oncology, Leeds Cancer Centre, St James's University Hospital, Leeds Teaching Hospitals NHS Trust, Leeds

Dr Jane Younger, Consultant in Psychological Medicine, Clatterbridge Cancer Centre NHS Foundation Trust, Birkenhead

Dr Yin Zhou, GP and Clinical Research Fellow, Primary Care Unit, University of Cambridge, Cambridge

Dr Lucy Ziegler, Academic Fellow, Leeds Institute of Health Sciences, University of Leeds, Leeds

Preface

The great strides that have been made in cancer care and the technologies that surround cancer screening, diagnosis and treatment are important and well recognized. They have contributed to the radical improvements in cancer survivorship seen in recent decades across much of the world. It is, however, equally important to emphasize the advances that have been made in approaches to ensure that a person who is undergoing diagnostic investigations or cancer treatments, or who is a survivor of cancer, is kept at the centre of all activities. We have improved our knowledge of how to involve patients at all stages and ensure they achieve the best experience, well-being and quality of life. This book describes the progress we have made and the efforts that must continue to strengthen this patient-centred approach. In our attempts to do justice to this very broad subject, we have involved multi-professional teams as authors of both the perspective chapters and the case reports. The teams who have developed and edited this book, and who have written the individual contributions, include not only oncologists and patients but also psychologists, psychiatrists, nurses and allied health professionals, as well as a wide-ranging mixture of senior and junior people from the many professions.

To achieve the best patient-centred care, it is important to integrate the efforts of many disciplines, professions and institutions. Cancer care becomes increasingly complex and reaches across primary, secondary, tertiary and social care, requiring the interactions of many healthcare institutions in every sector. The importance of integrating specialized multidisciplinary cancer care through cancer networks and other arrangements has been recognized for more than two decades, but opportunities to improve integration and to ensure that it supports patient-centred care continue to grow. Perhaps most notably, modern health informatics provides us with excellent opportunities to integrate the care of cancer patients between disciplines, professions and institutions with the minimum of disruption to patients' lives. Increasingly, it will be possible to move information rather than patients around the healthcare system, allowing care to be delivered in an integrated way close to patients' homes for much of the time. Of course, important periods of time will continue to be needed in specialist facilities for the delivery of appropriate aspects of patient care.

This book is part of a prize-winning annual series of books on key topics in cancer care that are important to patients and professionals alike and that are growing, developing and shaping future approaches.

Galina Velikova, Lesley Fallowfield, Jane Younger, Ruth Board and Peter Selby, Editors
Johnathan Joffe, Chairman, Association of Cancer Physicians
Jane Maher, Joint Chief Medical Officer, Macmillan Cancer Support

Acknowledgements

Editors' acknowledgements

The editors and authors are grateful to all the patients who have inspired them to prepare this book and to work together to improve patient care.

The editors warmly acknowledge the support they have received in preparing the book. They are especially grateful to Macmillan Cancer Support for their sponsorship of the book and the workshop that preceded it, without which the whole project would not have been possible.

The editors, authors and publisher are most grateful to the Executive Committee of the Association of Cancer Physicians for their support and advice during the development of this book.

We are very grateful to Duncan Enright and Beverley Martin at EBN Health for their expert work, support, goodwill and interest in our purpose in preparing the book, and Nicole Goldman, who coordinated and oversaw the book's preparation and organization.

Professor Velikova would like to acknowledge the support of the University of Leeds and the Leeds Teaching Hospitals NHS Trust. Professor Fallowfield would like to acknowledge the support of the University of Sussex. Dr Younger would like to acknowledge the support of the Clatterbridge Cancer Centre NHS Foundation Trust. Dr Board would like to acknowledge the support of the University of Manchester and Lancashire Teaching Hospitals NHS Foundation Trust. Professor Selby would like to acknowledge the support of the University of Leeds and the Leeds Teaching Hospitals NHS Trust.

Galina Velikova, Lesley Fallowfield, Jane Younger, Ruth Board and Peter Selby

Association of Cancer Physicians

The *Problem Solving* series of cancer-related books is developed and prepared by the Association of Cancer Physicians, often in partnership with one or more other specialist medical organizations. As the representative body for medical oncologists in the UK, the Association of Cancer Physicians has a broad set of aims, including education for its own members and for non-members, including interested clinicians, healthcare professionals and the public. The *Problem Solving* series is a planned sequence of publications that derive from a programme of annual scientific workshops initiated in 2014 with 'Problem Solving in Acute Oncology' followed by 'Problem Solving in Older Cancer Patients', 'Problem Solving Through Precision Oncology' and, most recently, 'Problem Solving in Patient-Centred and Integrated Cancer Care'.

The publications involve considerable work from members and other contributors; this work is done without remuneration, as an educational service. The books have been well received and we are delighted with their standard. *Problem Solving in Older Cancer Patients* and *Problem Solving Through Precision Oncology* were awarded the BMA prizes for best oncology book of the year in 2016 and 2017, respectively.

The Association of Cancer Physicians wishes to thank all the contributors to this and previous books and to those yet to come.

Johnathan Joffe, Chairman, Association of Cancer Physicians

Abbreviations

ABVD	Doxorubicin, bleomycin, vinblastine, dacarbazine
ADT	Androgen deprivation therapy
AFP	Alpha-fetoprotein
Akt	Protein kinase B
ALK	Anaplastic lymphoma kinase
BRAF	Serine/threonine-protein kinase B-Raf
BSL	British Sign Language
CAM	Complementary and alternative medicine
CanCon	Joint Action on Cancer Control
CBT	Cognitive behavioural therapy
CCCN	Comprehensive cancer care network
CEA	Carcinoembryonic antigen
CK	Cytokeratin
CQUIN	Commissioning for quality and innovation
CRP	C-reactive protein
CRPC	Castrate-resistant prostate cancer
CTCAE	Common terminology criteria for adverse events
DART	Distress Assessment and Response Tool
dCRT	Definitive chemoradiotherapy
EGFR	Epidermal growth factor receptor
EPF	European Patients' Forum
ER	Oestrogen receptor
FDG	Fluorodeoxyglucose
FIGO	International Federation of Gynecology and Obstetrics
FISH	Fluorescence *in situ* hybridization
FOLFOX	Fluorouracil, folinic acid, oxaliplatin
GCSF	Granulocyte-colony stimulating factor
hCG	Human chorionic gonadotrophin
HER2	Human epidermal growth factor receptor 2
HNA	Holistic needs assessment
HRQOL	Health-related quality of life
IVADO	Ifosfamide, vincristine, dactinomycin, doxorubicin
LDH	Lactate dehydrogenase
LHRHa	Luteinizing hormone-releasing hormone analogue
MAPK	Mitogen-activated protein kinase
MDT	Multidisciplinary team
MEK	Mitogen-activated protein kinase kinase
NCSI	National Cancer Survivorship Initiative
NSCLC	Non-small-cell lung carcinoma
OxMdG	Oxaliplatin, fluorouracil, folinic acid
pCR	Pathological complete response
PD-L1	Programmed death-ligand 1
PPIE	Patient and public involvement and engagement
PR	Progesterone receptor
PROMs	Patient-reported outcome measures
PS	Performance status
PSA	Prostate-specific antigen
QOL	Quality of life
RANKL	Receptor activator of nuclear factor kappa-B ligand
SACT	Systemic anticancer therapy
SDI-21	21-item Social Difficulties Inventory
TKI	Tyrosine kinase inhibitor
TPN	Total parenteral nutrition
TTF-1	Thyroid transcription factor 1
TYA	Teenage and young adult
VIDE	Vincristine, ifosfamide, doxorubicin, etoposide

We would like to dedicate the book to
Mike Baum, Ken Calman, Jim Till and Peter Maguire.

01 Patient-Centred and Integrated Cancer Care

Peter Selby, Ruth E. Board, Galina Velikova

Introduction

The delivery of cancer care must focus on ensuring the best outcomes and experience for the patient by drawing on the wide range of skills of the multidisciplinary team (MDT). These are a combination of clinical and technical skills, together with good communication, empathy and involvement of the patient in all aspects of care planning and delivery. Patient-centred care necessitates excellence in the quality and speed of diagnostic work and in the delivery of treatment, follow-up and long-term support. It requires control of the tumour and the best possible patient survival. We must also optimize health-related quality of life (HRQOL), patient experience and patient satisfaction with care. The best clinical options should be identified, preferably by a specialized MDT. The options are then considered with the patient, the family and carers. Decisions must take into account the views of both the healthcare professionals and the patient. Delivering excellent patient-centred care requires good communication skills. Patient participation in shared decision making, patient empowerment, and patient engagement in individual care, service planning and research all contribute to driving excellent patient-centred care.

The terminology in this area is rightly constantly evolving. 'Patient-centred care' is widely used to describe these aspects of cancer care, and we have used the term in this book. We recognize, however, that as the field extends to include approaches to people who undergo screening tests and diagnostic investigations, and as cancer survivors take up the reins of their lives again, the term 'person-centred care' becomes increasingly appropriate. This book brings together colleagues from a wide range of healthcare disciplines to articulate their understanding of patient-centred care, how to deliver it and how to consolidate its position in cancer care systems. A key aspect of developing and delivering excellent patient-centred care is the collaboration between many professions and disciplines. Integration of care can improve outcomes for cancer patients and is especially important to ensure a patient-centred approach.

Commitments to patient-centred care have been in place for several decades. An early example in the UK lay in the 1995 Calman–Hine report,[1] which said: 'The development of cancer services should be patient-centred and should take account of patients', families' and carers' views and preferences as well as those of professionals involved in cancer care. Individuals' perceptions of their needs may differ from those of the professional. Good communication between professionals and patients is especially important.' These concepts are brought up to date and elegantly expressed by Abrahams *et al.*[2] (Figure 1.1).

Key challenges

Excellence in patient-centred care has many challenges. Patient outcomes have many aspects, and assessing them requires increasingly complex outcome measures, often patient-reported outcome measures (PROMs) (see Chapter 2). Psychological and social factors are key aspects of patients'

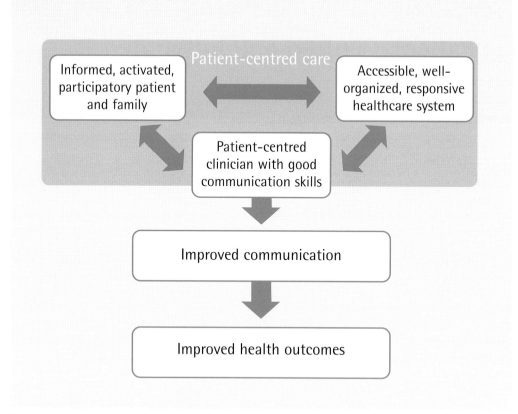

Figure 1.1 A model for patient-centred care (adapted from Abrahams et al.[2]).

quality of life (QOL) and require attention and measurement (see Chapters 2, 3 and 15). The training and skill set of the specialist oncology MDT must encompass high levels of communication skills; some team members will need advanced communication skills (see Chapter 4). The distribution of roles in the MDT will draw on different strengths to bring about a patient-centred approach. Some team members may be naturally excellent communicators; for others it will be an acquired skill. Teams should consciously plan their activities to draw on the strengths of their members. Increasingly, patient engagement and empowerment are contributing to improve the quality and outcomes of care (see Chapters 5 and 18). Primary care and the voluntary sector are vitally important in ensuring the best patient-centred care (see Chapters 6 and 7). As diagnosis and treatments improve, many more patients are surviving their cancers and require support during their periods of active treatment, as well as careful consideration of what is needed thereafter to ensure the best outcomes (see Chapters 8–12).

There is good evidence that cancer care can be delivered well when disciplines and institutions work together in an integrated way (see Chapter 13). However, we identify a series of special challenges to integrated cancer care. The first challenge is to integrate primary care and hospital care, which has been well reviewed by Rubin et al.[3] They concluded: 'The strengths of primary care – its continuous, coordinated, and comprehensive care for individuals and families – are particularly evident in prevention and diagnosis, in shared follow-up and survivorship care, and in end-of-life care.' Perhaps the greatest challenge for future links to primary care will come in the development of joint informatics approaches between primary care and the hospital oncology team to support communication between the teams and with patients that will underpin speed and excellence. These developments will aid improvements in GP–oncology MDT communications that will support work on earlier cancer diagnosis, patients' whole cancer journey, and integrated hospital–community approaches to survivorship and rehabilitation (see Chapters 8–13).

Second, links between oncology and palliative care have always been central to the best patient-centred approaches; these have been reviewed recently by Hui and Bruera.[4] The integration of palliative and supportive care throughout the patient's journey will bring well-recognized benefits in terms of QOL, symptom control and patient experience (see Chapters 11 and 12). There is emerging evidence that early palliative care can be associated with improved service delivery and possibly improved survival.[5]

Third, links between oncology and geriatrics will be vitally important.[6] Cancer is a disease of older people and in the UK two-thirds of our patients are diagnosed when over the age of 65 years. In general, older people are diagnosed later, have less treatment and their cure rates are generally lower. The reasons underpinning the low uptake of major cancer treatments in older people are poorly defined, but probably include comorbidity as well as patient preference and healthcare professional biases.

Fourth, the best outcomes for patients, including the best QOL and the best experience, mean that the specialist oncology team must link with other hospital disciplines to bring in their skills during both the diagnosis and management of their patients. Modern health informatics is increasingly facilitating such links and approaches. Electronic patient records enable good communications between hospital teams to the benefit of patients (see Chapter 13).

Finally, and importantly, close liaison between psychology, psychiatry, GPs, social services and cancer specialists is essential to achieve excellent, integrated, patient-centred care.

Patient-centred care acknowledges patients' individual information needs and the need for support for both physical and psychological health. It is important to recognize and adapt patient-centred care depending on the individual patient's wishes, background, social support and physical and psychological comorbidities. Integrating with a range of other medical specialties, allied healthcare professionals and third sector providers such as charitable organizations can help tailor communication and treatment for individual patient needs.

Tools to promote patient–centred care

A substantial number of tools need to be deployed to ensure that the care of cancer patients is both excellent and patient-centred.

- Clear policy and guidance on the importance and best ways to achieve patient-centred care.[7–11] Commissioners and management models should specify patient-centred approaches.
- An emphasis on patient-centred approaches in healthcare professionals' training and in the leadership, organization and management of health services.
- Patient engagement and empowerment (see Chapter 5) are powerful sources of influence on care quality. We should consistently seek patient input. Initiatives can be 'co-produced' by patients and healthcare professionals. As we develop new policies and plans, joint working between healthcare professionals and patients, carers and advocates will ensure a patient-centred approach.[8]

- Excellence in communication training for healthcare professionals.
- Provision of ongoing holistic needs assessment and support for patients by front line healthcare professionals and appropriate engagement of specialized psychosocial oncology services and counselling.
- Modern health informatics can ensure ready communications and access to information for patients and healthcare professionals and will underpin the future of patient-centred care.
- Measuring HRQOL and PROMs in clinical practice, clinical research and population studies (see Chapter 2). Such measurements provide insights into patient well-being, experience and quality of outcome, as well as valuable quantitative feedback on the attainment of patient-centred goals. The ability to measure QOL through PROMs allows us to draw attention to these key issues and measure the impact of efforts to provide excellent patient-centred care.

Conclusion

There is a longstanding consensus that cancer care should be patient-centred and integrated and there is considerable agreement about what that means. There is recognition, however, that patient-centred and integrated care is difficult to achieve and remains incomplete, but we have powerful tools to support continued progress. The chapters and case studies in this book provide evidence, advice and guidance to help healthcare professionals achieve these aims.

References

1 Calman K, Hine D. *A policy framework for commissioning cancer services. A report by the Expert Advisory Group on Cancer to the chief medical officers of England and Wales.* London: Department of Health, 1995.

2 Abrahams E, Foti M, Kean MA. Accelerating the delivery of patient-centered, high-quality cancer care. *Clin Cancer Res* 2015; 21: 2263–7.

3 Rubin G, Berendsen A, Crawford SM, *et al.* The expanding role of primary care in cancer control. *Lancet Oncol* 2015; 16: 1231–72.

4 Hui D, Bruera E. Models of integration of oncology and palliative care. *Ann Palliat Med* 2015; 4: 89–98.

5 Temel JS, Greer JA, Muzikansky A, *et al.* Early palliative care for patients with metastatic non-small-cell lung cancer. *N Engl J Med* 2010; 363: 733–42.

6 Ring A, Harari D, Kalsi T, *et al.*, eds. *Problem solving in older cancer patients.* Oxford: Clinical Publishing, 2015.

7 The Independent Cancer Taskforce (2015). *Achieving world-class cancer outcomes: a strategy for England 2015–2020.* Available from: www.cancerresearchuk.org/sites/default/files/achieving_world-class_cancer_outcomes_-_a_strategy_for_england_2015-2020.pdf (accessed 26 July 2017).

8 Lawler M, Banks M, Law K, *et al.* The European Cancer Patient's Bill of Rights, update and implementation 2016. *ESMO Open* 2016; 1: e000127.

9 Martin-Moreno JM, Albreht T, Radoš Krnel S, eds. *Boosting innovation and cooperation in European cancer control. Key findings from the European Partnership for Action against Cancer.* Ljubljana: National Institute of Public Health of the Republic of Slovenia; Brussels: World Health Organization, on behalf of the European Observatory on Health Systems and Policies, 2013.

10 Albreht T, Kiasuwa T, Van den Bulcke M, eds. *European guide on quality improvement in comprehensive cancer control.* Ljubljana: National Institute of Public Health of the Republic of Slovenia; Brussels: Scientific Institute of Public Health, 2017.

11 Federici A, Nicoletti G, Van den Bulcke M, eds. *Cancer control joint action policy papers.* Ljubljana: National Institute of Public Health of the Republic of Slovenia; Brussels: Scientific Institute of Public Health, 2017

02 Monitoring of Symptoms, Toxicity and Functioning Using Patient-Reported Outcome Measures

Alexandra Gilbert, Peter Selby, Galina Velikova

Introduction

Robust assessment of cancer patients' physical symptoms, the side effects of treatment and their impact on daily functioning and well-being is essential for modern oncology practice. Many cancer treatments have a narrow therapeutic range with often significant toxicity and small clinical benefits. The traditional medical interview to elicit symptoms and the formal recording of adverse events in clinical trials using the Common Terminology Criteria for Adverse Events (CTCAE) can be supplemented by structured symptom and functional information derived directly from patients.

Patient-reported outcome measures (PROMs) are defined as 'any report of the status of a patient's health condition that comes directly from the patient, without interpretation of the patient's response by a clinician or anyone else'.[1] PROMs provide a formal measurement of the subjective phenomena that make up the patient's perception of symptoms, daily functioning and health-related quality of life (HRQOL) and they carry important information on care quality. They can be measured using carefully developed and validated questionnaires. These measures can be applied in clinical trials to compare patient outcomes, in routine oncology practice to support patient care, and in population surveys.

The first PROMs used in oncology were HRQOL questionnaires. These multidimensional questionnaires measure physical symptoms, psychological distress, the impact on daily functioning and patient perceptions of their quality of life (QOL) and well-being.[2–5] More recently, a movement towards including patient voices in drug safety evaluations has focused on robust assessment of physical symptoms and side effects in clinical trials. This led to the development by the National Cancer Institute of a patient-reported outcomes version of the CTCAE system, known as the PRO-CTCAE.[6] In parallel, aspirations to provide better patient-centred care recommended PROMs for holistic needs assessment of all cancer patients, using screening tools such as the Distress Thermometer and Concerns Checklist.

PROMs in oncology trials

Traditionally PROMs, specifically HRQOL questionnaires, have been used in oncology trials as secondary outcome measures in addition to cancer outcomes such as overall or progression-free survival. This approach provided valuable information on side effects and patients' experiences with new treatments. Systematic reviews show that the measurement of HRQOL supported clinical decision making in a range of clinical trials.[7]

In an important recent example, the Prostate Testing for Cancer and Treatment (ProtecT) trial randomized 1643 men diagnosed by prostate-specific antigen levels to active monitoring, radical surgery or radiotherapy. PROMs were collected on urinary, bowel and sexual functions, and their effects on QOL. Urinary and sexual functioning were better in patients managed by active monitoring or radiotherapy (Figure 2.1), but general HRQOL scores were equivalent.[8] Given that the 10 year survival was equivalent, robust PROMs data will have a major influence on shared decision making, patient management and policy.

From a broader perspective, the formal assessment of HRQOL in oncology trials in past decades has brought patient well-being into risk–benefit considerations when recommending cancer treatments and has contributed to a recognition of the importance of patient-centred care and shared decision making.

PROMs in routine clinical care

With the wider use of electronic methods for data collection and electronic medical records, it has become feasible to collect PROMs in daily oncology practice and use them in real time to support individual patient care. PROMs data may be collected as a screening tool for symptoms or psychological distress, and used for monitoring symptoms and treatment response over time. Feeding back PROMs data in a structured format to the clinician can promote patient-centred care by highlighting concerns and prompting discussions. A number of randomized clinical trials that studied the use of PROMs in the routine care of cancer patients during treatment showed that providing PROMs to oncology clinicians can help identify psychological and physical problems, facilitate patient–doctor communication, engage patients in decision making, and

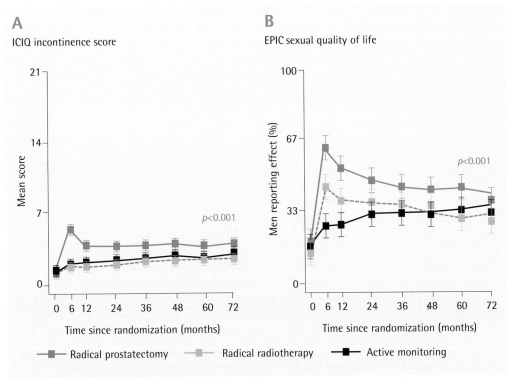

Figure 2.1 Example of use of PROMs data in the ProtecT trial. (A) Patient-reported effect of treatment on continence. (B) Patient-reported effect of treatment on sexual QOL. EPIC, Expanded Prostate Cancer Index Composite; ICIQ, International Consultation on Incontinence Questionnaire. Higher scores on each scale indicate worse symptoms or QOL. (Adapted from Donovan et al.[8])

Table 2.1 Overview of randomized controlled trials using PROMs in oncology practice.

Reference	Patient sample (n)	Communication	Patient well-being
McLachlan et al.[9]	450	NA	Reduction in depression
Detmar et al.[10]	214	+	–
Velikova et al.[11]	286	+	Improved HRQOL
Rosenbloom et al.[12]	213	+/–	–
Carlson et al.[13]	585	+	Reduced distress
Berry et al.[14]	660	+	NA
Berry et al.[15]	752	NA	Reduced distress
Basch et al.[16]	766	NA	Improved HRQOL Fewer emergency visits

NA, not applicable.

improve symptom control and patient well-being (Table 2.1). Two recent systematic reviews of the 25 randomized controlled trials in this field have been conducted.[17,18] Chen et al.[17] concluded: 'Despite the existence of significant gaps in the evidence base, there is growing evidence in support of routine PROM collection in enabling better and patient-centred care in cancer settings.'

In a randomized controlled trial performed in Leeds, using touchscreen computers in outpatient clinics, we allocated patients on chemotherapy for advanced cancer to one of three groups: (1) an HRQOL intervention group completed an HRQOL questionnaire in clinic and the scores were fed back to the oncologist; (2) an attention-control group completed an HRQOL questionnaire in clinic but the scores were not fed back; or (3) a usual care group. We observed a positive impact on communication, better control of symptoms and improved patient well-being over time in the HRQOL intervention group.[11] Figure 2.2A shows that a larger proportion of patients in the HRQOL intervention group (40%) had a clinically meaningful improvement in well-being in comparison with the other groups. These results are remarkably similar to those of a recent clinical trial performed in the USA that implemented web-based symptom self-reporting based on CTCAE during advanced cancer treatment.[16] Figure 2.2B shows that 34% of patients in the symptom-reporting group had improvement in the EuroQol five dimensions questionnaire, compared with 18% in the group that received usual care. Importantly, a reduced number of emergency room visits was also observed.

A further extension of the research in this area has been the development of electronic patient reporting of adverse events. Electronic Patient Self-Reporting of Adverse Events: Patient Information and Advice (eRAPID) is an online system for PROMs monitoring during and after cancer treatment. It has the ambitious aim to improve the safe delivery of cancer treatments, enhance patient care and standardize documentation of side effects in the clinical datasets. eRAPID allows patients to self-report symptoms and side effects, from home or hospital, with immediate real-time integration of results for display in existing electronic patient records, enabling the reports to be used in routine care. An innovative clinical algorithm, developed with clinicians, generates alerts for severe symptoms to the relevant clinical team or provides patient advice on managing mild symptoms (Figure 2.3). An ongoing programme funded by the National Institute for Health Research is evaluating the eRAPID approach during systemic therapy in a randomized controlled trial, and in pilot studies during and after radiotherapy and after upper gastrointestinal

A

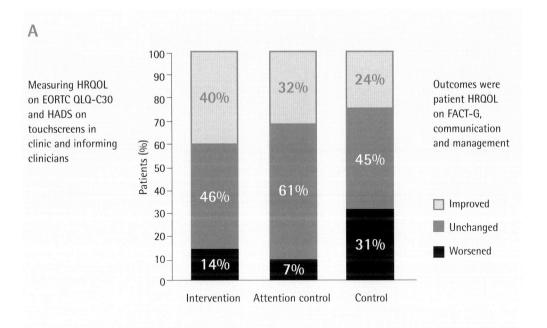

Measuring HRQOL on EORTC QLQ-C30 and HADS on touchscreens in clinic and informing clinicians

Outcomes were patient HRQOL on FACT-G, communication and management

B

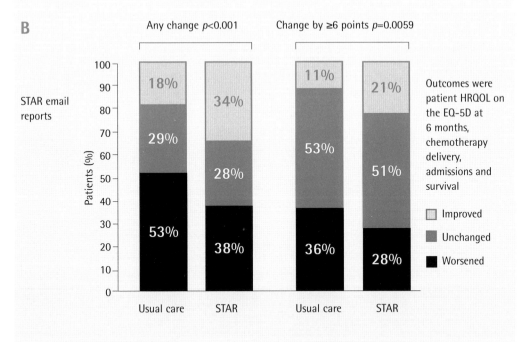

STAR email reports

Outcomes were patient HRQOL on the EQ-5D at 6 months, chemotherapy delivery, admissions and survival

Figure 2.2 Proportions of patients showing clinically meaningful improvement, no change, or worsening in their well-being when PROMs are used to monitor cancer patients during treatment. (A) Changes in Functional Assessment of Cancer-General (FACT-G) scores (adapted from Velikova et al.[11]). (B) Changes in EuroQol five dimensions questionnaire (EQ-5D) scores (adapted from Basch et al.[16]). EORTC, European Organisation for Research and Treatment of Cancer; HADS, Hospital Anxiety and Depression Scale.

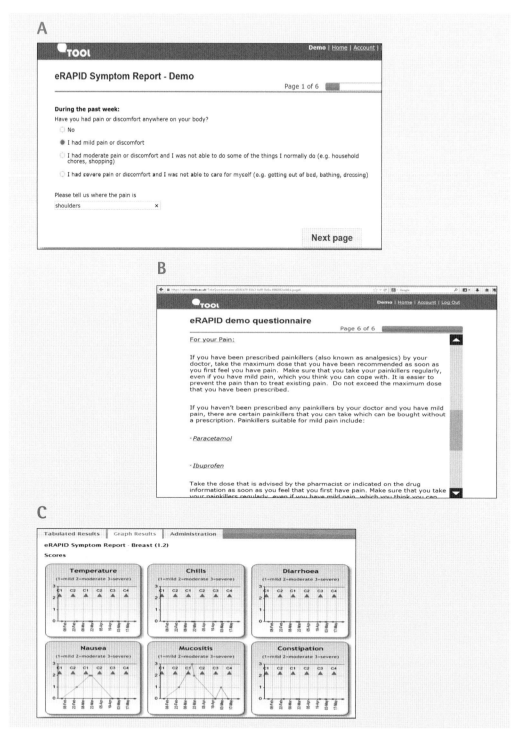

Figure 2.3 (A) Patient view of symptom self-reports. (B) Automated advice for mild symptoms. (C) Clinician view of symptom reports in electronic patient records in real time.

surgery. Case 14 and Case 19 give examples of how the eRAPID system is used to implement PROMs in routine patient care for symptom monitoring during and after radiotherapy treatment, and as part of an innovative model for remote follow-up of testicular cancer patients.

In order to move the field beyond clinical research and into routine patient care, international organizations such as the International Society for Quality of Life Research and the Quality of Life Group of the European Organisation for Research and Treatment of Cancer have developed practical guidelines on how to incorporate PROMs in clinical practice.[19,20] Patient education is recommended to support online reporting, along with an ethical responsibility to provide patients with clear guidance and advice on managing symptoms and alerting their clinical team about severe adverse symptoms. Training healthcare professionals in how to interpret PROMs scores and how to integrate them into their routine care is also of paramount importance.[21] A number of successful training approaches exist, but they have to be adapted to local needs and cultures. Using organization-wide approaches to change management and innovation will be needed to make PROMs a reality in clinical care.[22]

An excellent example of successful large-scale implementation of PROMs (>40,000 patient reports collected over the past 10 years) is the Interactive Symptom Assessment and Collection (ISAAC) system of Cancer Care Ontario, Canada, which was recently superseded by the Improving the Patient Experience and Health Outcomes Collaborative (iPEHOC) toolkit. Other examples of successful implementation of electronic PROMs systems include PatientViewpoint, the Computer-based Health Evaluation System (CHES), and the Symptom Tracking and Reporting System (STAR) (for an overview, see Jensen *et al.*[23]). In the UK and EU, the Advanced Symptom Management System (ASyMS) mobile phone system is being evaluated. Electronic PROMs systems have proven very acceptable even for patients coping with extreme symptom burden and reduced QOL.

PROMs population surveys

In 2008 the Darzi report recommended that collection of PROMs data should be an essential component of healthcare evaluation.[24] Nationwide use of PROMs began in elective surgical procedures, particularly for performance comparisons.

The first national pilot study of cancer survivors' experiences was conducted in 2015, establishing the feasibility of this approach and providing data on long-term consequences of treatment by cancer and treatment types.[25] The Life after a Prostate Cancer Diagnosis (LAPCD) project surveyed 60,000 prostate cancer survivors in the UK and achieved a 60% response rate, including 85% of NHS trusts in England and all NHS trusts in Wales, Scotland and Northern Ireland. Such a response rate demonstrates the feasibility of using PROMs on a population basis, and improvements in health informatics will make this approach generally accessible.[26]

In 2015, the Independent Cancer Taskforce report *Achieving world-class cancer outcomes* made a recommendation to NHS England to develop a national metric on QOL to enable better evaluation of long-term effects of cancer treatment in order to improve outcomes.[27] Large-scale data collection is planned to commence in 2018 with an aspiration to implement electronic PROMs collection to enable immediate use of the PROMs data in individual patient care (where appropriate), as well as for a performance quality indicator.

Conclusion

The development of health informatics has made the routine collection and use of PROMs possible in cancer care. The integration of PROMs with electronic patient records and the provision of advice based on algorithms can facilitate supported self-management of mild symptoms and timely hospital admissions for serious symptoms. Future work is likely to focus on the effectiveness of PROMs in longer term follow-up and on the increased use of mobile devices.

Standardized reporting of the combined clinical and PROMs data will help clinicians and providers to evaluate treatment benefits from the patient perspective, collect information on late effects of treatments and potentially measure the benefit of rehabilitation interventions. Pooled data with cancer registries, large clinical datasets and PROMs will incorporate cancer survivors' perspectives into the big data concept to inform improvements in healthcare and policy.

References

1 Food and Drug Administration (2009). *Guidance for industry. Patient-reported outcome measures: use in medical product development to support labeling claims.* Available from: www.fda.gov/downloads/drugs/guidances/ucm193282.pdf (accessed 1 May 2017).

2 Priestman TJ, Baum M. Evaluation of quality of life in patients receiving treatment for advanced breast cancer. *Lancet* 1976; 1: 899–900.

3 Selby P, Chapman JA, Etazadi-Amoli J, *et al.* The development of a method for assessing the quality of life of cancer patients. *Br J Cancer* 1984; 50: 13–22.

4 Aaronson NK, Ahmedzai S, Bergman B, *et al.* The European Organisation for Research and Treatment of Cancer QLQ-C30: a quality-of-life instrument for use in international clinical trials in oncology. *J Natl Cancer Inst* 1993; 85: 365–76.

5 Cella DF, Tulsky DS, Gray G, *et al.* The Functional Assessment of Cancer Therapy scale: development and validation of the general measure. *J Clin Oncol* 1993; 11: 570–9.

6 Basch E, Reeve BB, Mitchell SA, *et al.* Development of the National Cancer Institute's Patient-Reported Outcomes Version of the Common Terminology Criteria for Adverse Events (PRO-CTCAE). *J Natl Cancer Inst* 2014; 106: dju244.

7 Efficace F, Jacobs M, Pusic A, *et al.* Patient-reported outcomes in randomised controlled trials of gynaecological cancers: investigating methodological quality and impact on clinical decision-making. *Eur J Cancer* 2014; 50: 1925–41.

8 Donovan JL, Hamdy FC, Lane JA, *et al.* Patient-reported outcomes after monitoring, surgery, or radiotherapy for prostate cancer. *N Engl J Med* 2016; 375: 1425–37.

9 McLachlan SA, Allenby A, Matthews J, *et al.* Randomized trial of coordinated psychosocial interventions based on patient self-assessments versus standard care to improve the psychosocial functioning of patients with cancer. *J Clin Oncol* 2001; 19: 4117–25.

10 Detmar SB, Muller MJ, Wever LD, *et al.* The patient–physician relationship. Patient–physician communication during outpatient palliative treatment visits: an observational study. *JAMA* 2001; 285: 1351–7.

11 Velikova G, Booth L, Smith A, *et al.* Measuring quality of life in routine oncology practice improves communication and patient well-being: a randomized controlled trial. *J Clin Oncol* 2004; 22: 714–24.

12 Rosenbloom SK, Victorson DE, Hahn EA, *et al.* Assessment is not enough: a randomized controlled trial of the effects of HRQL assessment on quality of life and satisfaction in oncology clinical practice. *Psychooncology* 2007; 16: 1069–79.

13 Carlson LE, Groff SL, Maciejewski O, Bultz BD. Screening for distress in lung and breast cancer outpatients: a randomized controlled trial. *J Clin Oncol* 2010; 28: 4884–91.

14 Berry DL, Blumenstein BA, Halpenny B, *et al.* Enhancing patient–provider communication with the electronic self-report assessment for cancer: a randomized trial. *J Clin Oncol* 2011; 29: 1029–35.

15 Berry DL, Hong F, Halpenny B, *et al.* Electronic self-report assessment for cancer and self-care support: results of a multicenter randomized trial. *J Clin Oncol* 2014; 32: 199–205.

16 Basch E, Deal AM, Kris MG, *et al.* Symptom monitoring with patient-reported outcomes during routine cancer treatment: a randomized controlled trial. *J Clin Oncol* 2016; 34: 557–65.

17 Chen J, Ou L, Hollis SJ. A systematic review of the impact of routine collection of patient reported outcome measures on patients, providers and health organisations in an oncologic setting. *BMC Health Serv Res* 2013; 13: 211.

18 Kotronoulas G, Kearney N, Maguire R, *et al.* What is the value of the routine use of patient-reported outcome measures toward improvement of patient outcomes, processes of care, and health service outcomes in cancer care? A systematic review of controlled trials. *J Clin Oncol* 2014; 32: 1480–501.

19 Wintner LM, Sztankay M, Aaronson N, *et al.* The use of EORTC measures in daily clinical practice – a synopsis of a newly developed manual. *Eur J Cancer* 2016; 68: 73–81.

20 Snyder CF, Aaronson NK, Choucair AK, *et al.* Implementing patient-reported outcomes assessment in clinical practice: a review of the options and considerations. *Qual Life Res* 2012; 21: 1305–14.

21 Santana MJ, Haverman L, Absolom K, *et al.* Training clinicians in how to use patient-reported outcome measures in routine clinical practice. *Qual Life Res* 2015; 24: 1707–18.

22 Gilbert A, Sebag-Montefiore D, Davidson S, Velikova G. Use of patient-reported outcomes to measure symptoms and health related quality of life in the clinic. *Gynecol Oncol* 2015; 136: 429–39.

23 Jensen RE, Snyder CF, Abernethy AP, *et al.* Review of electronic patient-reported outcomes systems used in cancer clinical care. *J Oncol Pract* 2014; 10: e215-22.

24 Department of Health (2008). *High quality care for all. NHS next stage review final report.* Available from: www.gov.uk/government/uploads/system/uploads/attachment_data/file/228836/7432.pdf (accessed 3 July 2017).

25 Glaser AW, Fraser LK, Corner J, *et al.* Patient-reported outcomes of cancer survivors in England 1–5 years after diagnosis: a cross-sectional survey. *BMJ Open* 2013; 3: e002317.

26 Downing A, Wright P, Wagland R, *et al.* Life after prostate cancer diagnosis: protocol for a UK-wide patient-reported outcomes study. *BMJ Open* 2016; 6: e013555.

27 The Independent Cancer Taskforce (2015). *Achieving world-class cancer outcomes: a strategy for England 2015–2020.* Available from: www.cancerresearchuk.org/sites/default/files/achieving_world-class_cancer_outcomes_-_a_strategy_for_england_2015-2020.pdf (accessed 3 July 2017).

03 Assessment of Psychological Distress in Cancer

Jane Younger

Introduction

A diagnosis of cancer affects every aspect of a person's life. It can be like a bomb going off, damaging not only the area affected, but everything around it: from physical health to psychological well-being; from social functioning to financial stability. Like a bomb, some effects are immediate but others may not appear for some time. It is the immediate effects that are treated in the first instance, but the other damage can harm the foundations of lives and relationships. The effect is not limited to the person with the disease but also spreads to those around them.

It was suggested by Dr Adam Glaser at the Kings Fund conference in 2013 on patient-reported outcome measures[1] that patients have three questions: Will I survive? Will I be well looked after? What will I be like? Immediately after diagnosis, most patients' main concern is with the first question, 'Will I survive?' Frequently, this is the first time a patient will have had to contemplate his or her mortality. Typically, patients experience shock and a period of turmoil which affect their sleep, appetite and day-to-day functioning. This usually diminishes over time, and the focus moves to treatment, which can be gruelling and consumes most of the patient's physical and emotional energy. It is often only when treatment is finished that there is the emotional energy to think about the last question, 'What will I be like?', which is when thoughts develop about what a diagnosis of cancer means to them, to their family and to their future.

Prevalence of psychological distress and psychiatric disorder

'Psychological distress' is a term which includes symptoms such as worry, intrusive thoughts, low mood, poor concentration, sleep difficulties and appetite changes, but which may be below the threshold for a diagnosable psychiatric condition. Psychological distress becomes clinically significant when it begins to impact a person's life: in patients with cancer the prevalence of mental disorder has been shown to be between 30% and 40%.[2] The most common mental disorders are adjustment, depression and anxiety disorders.[2] Studies examining the prevalence of major depressive illness show figures varying from 8%[3] to around 25%,[4] and the prevalence of anxiety disorder to be about 25%.[4] In 2013 a systematic review of the prevalence of depression in adults with cancer concluded that rates are imprecise due to differences in study design; however, it is clear that psychological morbidity is a significant part of the cancer diagnosis for many people.[5]

Current recommendations for psychological support

In 2004 NICE issued guidance on improving supportive and palliative care for adults with cancer.[6] It recommended that psychological support should be provided in a stepped care approach which addresses the needs of patients with few psychological needs through to those needing specific intervention (Table 3.1). It recommended that every member of the

Table 3.1 Recommended model of professional psychological assessment and support.[6]

Level	Who should provide it?	What should be assessed?	What is the intervention?
1	All health and social care professionals	Recognition of psychological needs	Effective information giving, compassionate communication and general psychological support
2	Health and social care professionals with additional expertise (including CNS)	Screening for psychological distress	Use of standardized screening tools, e.g. the Distress Thermometer and the Hospital Anxiety and Depression Scale
3	Trained and accredited professionals	Assessments for psychological distress and diagnosis of some psychopathology	Counselling and specific psychological interventions such as anxiety management and solution-focused therapy, delivered according to an explicit therapeutic framework
4	Mental health specialists	Diagnosis of psychopathology	Specialist psychological and psychiatric interventions such as psychotherapy, including cognitive behavioural therapy

CNS, clinical nurse specialist.

multidisciplinary team (MDT) should be able to recognize patients' psychological needs and be able to communicate effectively and with compassion (level 1).

Level 2 of the NICE guidance suggests that all patients should be screened for psychological morbidity at key points in their disease, which include around the time of diagnosis, during treatment, as treatment ends, and at the time of disease recurrence. Oncology teams are poor at recognizing psychological distress: Fallowfield et al.[7] showed that 36.4% of screened patients had scores suggesting psychiatric morbidity, but doctors picked up less than one-third of these cases. A smaller scale study in 2016 similarly showed that a group of newly diagnosed patients attending for radiotherapy commonly had symptoms of psychological distress (and depression and anxiety) but that these were infrequently addressed.[8]

NICE recommends that each MDT should have at least one member who has additional psychological skills to assess psychological distress and provide psychological support. This person should have level 2 psychological skills training, also known as holistic needs assessment (HNA) training, and should join a monthly supervision group to help consolidate their skills and give them support in approaching what can often be challenging topics. This role is usually done by the clinical nurse specialist, but it can be done by any member of the MDT.

For most patients presenting with psychological distress, recognition of their difficulties, and eliciting and addressing their concerns, is the only intervention needed. Some patients may require more support than their oncology team can offer and in these cases signposting to third sector support services can be very helpful. Some patients may have more significant psychological morbidity and need referral to specialist psychological support services. Level 3 psychological support is counselling or a specific psychological therapy provided by a therapist with experience of working in cancer. Level 4 is assessment and treatment by a mental health professional who works in cancer care; this level of support is provided by clinical psychology or liaison psychiatry services.

Assessment of psychological need

Since the NICE guidance in 2004 there has been discussion as to how psychological distress should best be assessed. Tools including the Hospital Anxiety and Depression Scale[9] and the Distress Thermometer[10] have been suggested. However, the majority of patients continue not to be screened: reasons for this include lack of time as well as uncertainty as to how to screen and fear of being unable to deal with the patient's concerns.[11]

The National Cancer Survivorship Initiative (NCSI), which was launched in 2007, made a number of recommendations including a shift towards HNA and self-management. The *Living with and beyond cancer* paper[12] produced by the Department of Health and Macmillan Cancer Support in 2013 took forward the NCSI vision and suggested that all patients should have a treatment summary, an HNA, a written care plan, and advice on rehabilitation and healthy living. Macmillan Cancer Support developed an HNA tool which could be used not just at the end of treatment but throughout a patient's journey to fulfil the level 2 psychological support required by NICE guidance.

HNA

Developed by Macmillan Cancer Support to systematically identify the patient's needs to enable him or her to live well with cancer, it was hoped that routine assessment of all patients would reveal the needs of the population. The HNA (Figure 3.1) is completed by the patient and used as the basis for discussion with a health professional (usually someone with level 2 psychological skills) who can then identify any areas of concern with the patient and develop a care plan to address them. Initially the HNA was on paper but an electronic version, the eHNA, was launched in 2012 and since then over 17,000 care plans have been developed.[13] Data about concerns elicited on the eHNA combined with clinical information have been used to create an anonymized database of care plans held on a secure NHS network, allowing information about patients' main concerns and difficulties to be examined on a large scale. This electronic assessment is most commonly completed at diagnosis. The biggest limitation to its completion is time; in addition, some high-need patients are not thought to be eligible for HNA; also, clinicians are concerned that they may not be able to deal with the concerns expressed.[11]

In 51% of eHNA assessments, no concerns were expressed and in 12% only one concern was expressed.[13] The two most common concerns are worry, fear and anxiety, and fatigue, both expressed by 12.8% of the patients who had an HNA, followed by pain (7.7%) and sleep problems (7.4%).[13] Some patterns of concerns have been noted. Fatigue, pain, and worry, fear and anxiety are often expressed together, as are sleep problems, memory and concentration, and worry, fear and anxiety. Concerns grouped like this may indicate a depressive illness or an anxiety disorder that needs further assessment.

It is important that the assessment is shared with the whole treating team so that they can be aware of the patient's concerns and difficulties, as these can affect consultations and the choices made by the patient, and it may be that other team members can suggest alternative ways to move forward.

National Cancer Survivorship Initiative – Concerns checklist   Holistic needs assessment

Identifying your concerns

Patient's name or label

Discussed by: _____

Date: _____

Designation: _____

Contact details: _____

This self–assessment is optional; however, it will help us understand the concerns and feelings you have. It will also help us identify any information and support you may need in the future.

If any of the problems below have caused you concern in the past week and if you wish to discuss them with a healthcare professional, please tick the box. Leave the box blank if it doesn't apply to you or you don't want to discuss it now.

☐ I have questions about my diagnosis/treatment that I would like to discuss.

Physical concerns
☐ Breathing difficulties
☐ Passing urine
☐ Constipation
☐ Diarrhoea
☐ Eating or appetite
☐ Indigestion
☐ Sore or dry mouth
☐ Nausea or vomiting
☐ Sleep problems/nightmares
☐ Tired/exhausted or fatigued
☐ Swollen tummy or limb
☐ High temperature or fever
☐ Getting around (walking)
☐ Tingling in hands/feet
☐ Pain
☐ Hot flushes/sweating
☐ Dry, itchy or sore skin
☐ Wound care after surgery
☐ Changes in weight
☐ Memory or concentration
☐ Taste/sight/hearing
☐ Speech problems
☐ My appearance
☐ Sex/intimacy/fertility

Practical concerns
☐ Caring responsibilities
☐ Work and education
☐ Money or housing
☐ Insurance and travel
☐ Transport or parking
☐ Contact/communication
    with NHS staff
☐ Laundry/housework
☐ Washing and dressing
☐ Preparing meals/drinks
☐ Grocery shopping

Family/relationship concerns
☐ Partner
☐ Children
☐ Other relatives/friends

Emotional concerns
☐ Difficulty making plans
☐ Loss of interest/activities
☐ Unable to express feelings
☐ Anger or frustration
☐ Guilt
☐ Hopelessness
☐ Loneliness or isolation
☐ Sadness or depression
☐ Worry, fear or anxiety

Spiritual or religious concerns
☐ Loss of faith or other
    spiritual concerns
☐ Loss of meaning
    or purpose of life
☐ Not being at peace with
    or feeling regret about the past

Lifestyle or information needs
☐ Support groups
☐ Complementary therapies
☐ Diet and nutrition
☐ Exercise and activity
☐ Smoking
☐ Alcohol or drugs
☐ Sun protection
☐ Hobbies
☐ Staying in/returning to
    work and education
☐ Making a will
☐ Other

Please mark the scale to show the overall level of concern you've felt over the past week.

You may also wish to score the concerns you have ticked from 1 to 10.

1   10

Lowest   Highest

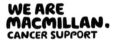

WE ARE
MACMILLAN.
CANCER SUPPORT

Figure 3.1 The NCSI HNA tool (reproduced by kind permission of Macmillan Cancer Support).

Conclusion

Patients with cancer have a high prevalence of psychological distress that often goes undetected by the clinical team. Screening tools may improve detection; nationally, there is a push for patients to have an HNA at key points during their disease trajectory. Barriers to using this tool may be the clinician's worry that it will take too long, or fear of not being able to help with the concerns expressed. Clinicians using the HNA or providing psychological support in other ways should have training and supervision to allow them to feel competent to deliver this care.

References

1 Glaser A (2013). *National cancer PROMS programme.* Available from: www.kingsfund.org.uk/sites/files/kf/media/adam-glaser-proms-cancer-survivors-dec13.pdf (accessed 7 June 2017).

2 Fischer D, Wedel B. Anxiety and depression disorders in cancer patients: incidence, diagnosis and therapy. *Memo Magazine Eur Med Oncol* 2012; 5: 52–4.

3 Sharpe M, Strong V, Allen K, *et al.* Major depression in outpatients attending a regional cancer centre: screening and unmet treatment needs. *Br J Cancer* 2004; 90: 314–20.

4 Decat CS, de Araujo TC, Nonino A, *et al.* Screening for psychological distress, anxiety and depression in cancer patients during the chemotherapy. *Psychooncology* 2009; 18 (suppl 2).

5 Walker J, Holm Hansen C, Martin P, *et al.* Prevalence of depression in adults with cancer: a systematic review. *Ann Oncol* 2013; 24: 895–900.

6 National Institute for Health and Clinical Excellence (2004). *Improving supportive and palliative care for adults with cancer.* Available from: www.nice.org.uk/guidance/csg4/resources/improving-supportive-and-palliative-care-for-adults-with-cancer-pdf-773375005 (accessed 15 June 2017).

7 Fallowfield L, Ratcliffe D, Jenkins V, Saul J. Psychiatric morbidity and its recognition by doctors in patients with cancer. *Br J Cancer* 2001; 84: 1011–15.

8 Silva RH, Gilani S, O'Donovan C. Assessment of psychological distress in cancer patients: a strong pillar for clinical interview. *Psychooncology* 2016; 25 (suppl 1).

9 Mitchell AJ, Meader N, Symonds P. Diagnostic validity of the Hospital Anxiety and Depression Scale (HADS) in cancer and palliative settings: a meta-analysis. *J Affect Disord* 2010; 126: 335–48.

10 Ma X, Zhang J, Zhong W, *et al.* The diagnostic role of a short screening tool – the Distress Thermometer: a meta-analysis. *Support Care Cancer* 2014; 22: 1741–55.

11 Ipsos Mori (2015). *Evaluation of the electronic holistic needs assessment (eHNA). Final evaluation report.* Available from: www.macmillan.org.uk/documents/aboutus/health_professionals/recoverypackage/macmillanehnafinalevaluationreport.pdf (accessed 13 June 2017).

12 Department of Health, Macmillan Cancer Support, NHS Improvement. *Living with and beyond cancer: taking action to improve outcomes.* London: Department of Health, 2013.

13 White R. A patient perspective analysis of electronic holistic needs assessment (eHNA). Presented at: National Cancer Registration and Analysis Service conference, Manchester, 13–14 June 2017. Poster.

04 Patient-Centred Decision Making: Communication Challenges

Lesley Fallowfield, Peter Selby

Introduction

Good communication is central to the provision of excellence in patient-centred care, especially when it underpins decisions and choices about diagnosis and treatment. Patient-centred approaches that depend on good communication are now built into the philosophy and culture and operational frameworks of the NHS and many healthcare services. NICE advises all NHS professionals to take into account individual needs and preferences. Patients should have the opportunity to make informed decisions about their care and treatment, in partnership with their healthcare professionals.[1] Similarly, the Institute of Medicine states that healthcare professionals should provide 'care that is respectful of and responsive to individual patient preferences, needs, and values and ensuring that patient values guide all clinical decisions'.[2] Patient-centred care is one of the seven core principles of NHS England.[3] Excellence in patient-centred care requires wise decision making following good communication and provision of good-quality information.

Good communication is a feature of every aspect of cancer care. Communication skills training is now part of undergraduate education in healthcare and of continuing professional education in all oncology disciplines. Advanced communication skills in cancer professionals bring benefits to cancer patients.[4,5] Many areas require training including breaking bad news[6] and explaining complex treatments and clinical trials. In all clinical settings, good communication begins with an ordinary, courteous introduction. Be sure that your patient knows who you are and what you are there to do. Tell the truth and try to listen as much as you talk. Beyond these social norms, however, an organized approach to communication is helpful.

The DREAM protocol to aid communication

The DREAM five-component protocol is a good example of an established communication approach with wide applicability (Table 4.1). It illustrates how a systematic approach can improve communications and add to the confidence of cancer professionals who face these challenges.[7]

Table 4.1 uses the DREAM outline to summarize the features of an approach to good communication with cancer patients. It is clear that patients usually want information about treatment options to be communicated carefully and honestly. There are increasing ethical, legal and social imperatives for patients to be more active and engaged in their care decisions and to be autonomous and collaborative rather than passive in decision making.[8] These imperatives are becoming arguably even more important now that so many complex treatment options exist for many cancer patients. Implicit in the term 'informed consent' is the idea that patients are told about the potential harms and benefits of different management plans including any appropriate alternative (such as clinical trial enrolment) and have the opportunity to ask questions about the logic and rationale behind any suggestions before they give their consent. Unfortunately, studies in the past 20 years across tumour sites have shown that there is often a mismatch between patients' understanding of information, their decision-making preferences and what actually occurs in clinical consultations.[9]

	Table 4.1 The DREAM interview: key components and skills needed.
Data	Collecting accurate data, i.e. taking a clear medical history needs knowledge about appropriate use of open, focused-open and closed questions, and avoidance of leading and multiple questions
	Set up the interview carefully and allow adequate time; include a patient's spouse, partner or friend who will help their recall; ensure you know the patient's pre-existing knowledge – their 'starting point'
Relationship	Establishing a relationship or rapport, i.e. learning more about the patient's worries and concerns and making the patient feel comfortable by giving and asking information, not interrupting too much or looking at notes
	This needs awareness of verbal and non-verbal communication and the ability to engage in active listening
Empathy	Being empathic, i.e. responding appropriately to patient-led cues Acknowledge the burden of disease and treatment
Advice	Giving advice, i.e. explaining the logic and rationale for treatment, and putting complex information into layperson's terms
	This needs the ability to structure information into manageable chunks, to summarize and to constantly check understanding.
	Encourage note taking or recordings: it is good practice to give patients brief notes of the main points at the end of the interview (these may be made by an accompanying healthcare professional)
Motivation	Providing motivation, i.e. ensuring that the patient understands the true therapeutic intent of treatment and feels motivated to embark on therapy with the likelihood of achieving realistic goals
	This needs use of unambiguous language and the ability to focus the patient on goals such as improving QOL

Decision-making preferences

Decision-making preferences are characterized in Figure 4.1. Identification of the 'best' approach in individual cases is often challenging and unclear. Patients who are unwell and anxious may find it difficult to convey their values and the background aspects of their lifestyle that will underpin their treatment preferences. The healthcare professionals involved in decision making hold considerable power as a result of their specialist knowledge. They do not usually have direct, personal experience of the consequences of the complex treatments that they describe to patients and subsequently deliver. Although shared decision making may be the desired goal for everyone, it is a challenging process particularly when clinicians have a strong view as to what might be in the patient's best interest or have been mandated by a multidisciplinary team with a clear preference. This preference may be right for the average patient but not necessarily right for every patient.[10] Nevertheless, it is important that we persevere in strengthening patient-centred approaches and good communication to reduce fear and anxiety. This should result in less regret about the decisions taken, enhance the patient's ability to employ coping strategies and ensure better compliance and adherence once joint decisions have been taken about management plans, all of which should ultimately lead to improved patient experience, better quality of life (QOL) and, through better adherence to treatment plans, improved survival.

The best patient-centred decision making must include giving information about therapeutic intent (cure, palliation) and all available options, as well as indicating what is involved: treatment

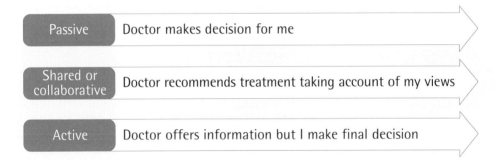

Figure 4.1 Decision-making preferences.

regimens and visits, scans and tests required. Clinicians need to elicit and understand the patient's perspectives (concerns, ideas, expectations), understand the patient within their unique psychosocial and cultural context and reach shared understanding about treatments concordant with the patient's values even though both parties might have competing agendas.

Owing to our better understanding of genetics and underlying cancer biology, which has facilitated many therapeutic advances in the past decade, the complexity of decision making in modern oncology must not be underestimated. We have multifarious improved diagnostics, surgical and radiotherapy techniques and better targeted systemic therapies, and more patients are surviving well and for longer; thus, cancer, which was never simple to explain, has now become even more complex. Furthermore, health and in particular statistical illiteracy are common and describing risks and benefits in terms of proportions and uncertainty is challenging.[10] Add to all this the fact that newly diagnosed patients experience emotional turmoil as they enter a strange new world of esoteric language and concepts and it becomes obvious why cancer professionals require adept communication skills to ensure that patients are able to provide truly educated/informed consent to treatments offered.

Approaches to how we best communicate ideas about treatment must begin with clarifying the patient's knowledge about cancer and its treatment. We can ask how much involvement in decision making is wanted at diagnosis and in the future; what is the patient's perception of a 'good' outcome from treatment; how can we help the patient be realistic about potential gains/harms; and how best should we handle relatives with different views.

The literature gives us insights into the characteristics of decision making. For instance, in a large study of US patients Keating *et al.*[11] observed some interesting differences: if patients showed strong evidence of personal efficacy then high levels of shared control were sought. The highest rates of patient control were seen in chemotherapy decisions; the highest rates of physician control were seen in surgery and radiation. We might expect patient preferences to predominate in settings where evidence of benefits is more modest and potential toxicity high, but this is not evident: results showed low patient and high physician control in such settings. This suggests that we need better strategies to engage patients when treatment is not curative.

Decision making by breast cancer patients

Decisions in the setting of breast cancer are complex. We know adherence rates to adjuvant endocrine therapy decline over time. Beryl *et al.*[12] mapped longitudinal decision-making processes in women, looking at patterns of uncertainty and decisional change over time. Surgery, intravenous systemic chemotherapy and radiotherapy decisions were seen as acute; oral medications, diet and exercise were fundamentally different, long-term decisions. Decisions on surgery were seen to be mainly irreversible and patients had a passive role during treatment. Oral medication compliance required active daily decisions by the patient and was reversible. In this setting the concept of decisional resolve is important and can change behaviour.

It is widely assumed that older patients may be less inclined to seek shared decision making and more deferential and passive. Ring *et al.*[13] found in older women (>70 years) that 18.9% wanted to make their own decision, 22.6% wanted to delegate decisions to the doctor and 58.5% preferred shared decision making. Their preferences had an influence on the acceptance of chemotherapy in that 50% of those wishing to make their own decision declined, as did 42.9% of those preferring shared decisions; patients who preferred their doctor to decide were more likely to accept chemotherapy.

Smith *et al.*[14] assessed the attitudes of women over 70 years of age towards surgery and neoadjuvant therapy for breast cancer. They worked in the setting of clear NICE guidelines:[15] 'Treat patients with early invasive breast cancer, irrespective of age, with surgery and appropriate systemic therapy, rather than endocrine therapy alone, unless significant comorbidity precludes surgery.' They surveyed 339 patients (192 mastectomy, 147 breast conservation) and investigated factors contributing to decisions. Most women expected that they would only be offered mastectomy; 18% of the mastectomy group would have preferred to have had breast-conserving surgery; 40% would have accepted neoadjuvant endocrine therapy to try and facilitate it; 86% of mastectomy patients said their surgeon had recommended the operation.[14]

The literature suggests that factors influencing the choice of surgery in early breast cancer are: perceived clinical outcomes, survival, fear of recurrence, treatment concerns/avoidance of radiotherapy, concern about appearance and body image, involvement in decision making, media reports, clinicians' preferences, perception of communication, and previous experiences and anticipations. A Cochrane review of 55 trials and 23 different screening/treatment decisions showed that greater knowledge and more accurate risk perceptions led to greater comfort with decisions and greater participation in decision making.[16]

Conclusion

We believe that patients want a good doctor–patient relationship: a doctor who is approachable and kind and provides respectful care. Patients want to explore thoughts, worries, feelings and expectations and have their input into decisions taken seriously. They need, and we should aim to provide, an understanding of how cancer affects a patient's life and family. Information needs to be uncomplicated, specific and unambiguous. Information should be delivered in an appropriate manner. Overly directive communication has negative consequences.

In delivering patient-centred care and improving communication with patients, healthcare professionals have a powerful influence on decision making; however, they are no longer the patient's only source of information. Clinical information and logic regarding treatment options may not be as salient to patients as healthcare professionals might think. Decisions are made in a process over time and involve other opinions, including those found on the internet and social media. Data about side effects that impact QOL and the burden of visits for scans, tests and treatment are not always available or factored into decisions. 'Doctor knows best' has resonance for some but not all patients. Communication is key to high-quality, patient-centred care.

References

1 National Institute for Health and Care Excellence (2012). *Patient experience in adult NHS services. Quality standard QS15.* Available from: www.nice.org.uk/guidance/qs15/resources/patient-experience-in-adult-nhs-services-2098486990789 (accessed 11 April 2017).

2 Institute of Medicine. *Crossing the quality chasm: a new health system for the 21st century.* Washington, DC: National Academies Press, 2001.

3 Department of Health (2012). *NHS Constitution for England. Principles and values that guide the NHS.* Available from: www.nhs.uk/NHSEngland/thenhs/about/Pages/nhscoreprinciples.aspx (accessed 11 April 2017).

4 Fallowfield L, Jenkins V, Farewell V, *et al.* Efficacy of a Cancer Research UK communication skills training model for oncologists: a randomised controlled trial. *Lancet* 2002; 359: 650–6.

5 Fallowfield L, Langridge C, Jenkins V. Communication skills training for breast cancer teams talking about trials. *Breast* 2014; 23: 193–7.

6 Payne J (2014). *Breaking bad news.* Available from: https://patient.info/doctor/breaking-bad-news (accessed 20 July 2017).

7 Fallowfield L, Jenkins V. Current concepts of communications skills training in oncology. *Recent Results Cancer Res* 2006; 168: 105–12.

8 Jenkins V, Fallowfield L, Saul J. Information needs of patients with cancer: results from a large study in UK cancer centres. *Br J Cancer* 2001; 84: 48–51.

9 Tariman JD, Berry DL, Cochrane B, *et al.* Preferred and actual participation roles during health care decision making in persons with cancer: a systematic review. *Ann Oncol* 2010; 21: 1145–51.

10 Gigerenzer G, Gaissmaier W, Kurz-Milcke E, *et al.* Helping doctors and patients make sense of health statistics. *Psychol Sci Public Interest* 2007; 8: 53–96.

11 Keating NL, Beth Landrum M, Arora NK, *et al.* Cancer patients' roles in treatment decisions: do characteristics of the decision influence roles? *J Clin Oncol* 2010; 28: 4364–70.

12 Beryl LL, Rendle KA, Halley MC, *et al.* Mapping the decision-making process for adjuvant endocrine therapy for breast cancer: the role of decisional resolve. *Med Decis Making* 2017; 37: 79–90.

13 Ring A, Harder H, Langridge C, *et al.* Adjuvant Chemotherapy in Elderly Women with Breast Cancer (AChEW): an observational study identifying MDT perceptions and barriers to decision making. *Ann Oncol* 2013; 24: 1211–19.

14 Smith LI, Dayal S, Murray J, Lannigan A. Attitudes towards breast conservation in patients aged over 70 with breast cancer. *Springerplus* 2016; 5: 478.

15 National Institute for Health and Care Excellence (2017). *Early and locally advanced breast cancer: diagnosis and treatment. Clinical guideline CG80.* Available from: www.nice.org.uk/guidance/cg80/chapter/1-guidance#primarysystemic-therapy (accessed 20 July 2017).

16 O'Connor AM, Bennett CL, Stacey D, *et al.* Decision aids for people facing health treatment or screening decisions. *Cochrane Database Syst Rev* 2009; 3: CD001431.

05 Patient Engagement and Empowerment: Key Components of Effective Patient-Centred Care

Hugh Butcher, Peter Selby

Introduction

The goals of patient-centred care require us to focus on the expressed needs and preferences of the patient, rather than on the needs and preferences of healthcare services or healthcare professionals. In this chapter we discuss the growing importance of patient engagement and patient empowerment, which for many patients represent two essential components of patient-centred care. Both engagement and empowerment stress that healthcare professionals and patients work in partnership to promote and support patients' active involvement in advancing their health and healthcare. The definitions used for these terms are not universally agreed but some clarity is emerging,[1] which is discussed in this chapter. It is useful to differentiate between the two terms. 'Engagement' expresses the commitment and actions of healthcare professionals to include patients in discussions and decisions about their care as individuals and in the development ('co-production') of plans for healthcare services. Patient engagement positively shapes the interactions between patients, healthcare professionals and healthcare services. 'Empowerment' is a wider, more complex concept that encompasses commitment and action by patients that are self-derived and self-driven and may occur outside the interactions with healthcare professionals. 'Engagement' and 'empowerment' overlap, interact and strengthen each other. The degree of empowerment or engagement that is desirable for an individual depends on the person's preferences and experience.

Engagement

Angela Coulter writes on patient engagement and comments that most patients want to play an active role in their healthcare: they want to know how to protect and improve their health when they are well; when they are ill, they want information about the treatment options and likely outcomes; and, in addition to seeking fast, effective health advice and care when they need it, most people want to know what they can do to help themselves.[2] Patient engagement therefore involves ensuring the following:

- Care delivery by healthcare professionals is always responsive to people's physical, emotional, social and cultural needs.
- Staff interactions with patients are empathetic and informative.
- The patient's personal values and preferences are elicited and acted upon.

The goal is to understand what matters most to patients, and that healthcare professionals re-orient service goals based on that understanding. This is well articulated in the UK on the INVOLVE website (www.invo.org.uk).

Empowerment

The European Patients' Forum (EPF) writes on patient empowerment and comments that it is defined in multiple ways depending on the context and objectives. The EPF defines empowerment as a 'process that helps people gain control over their own lives and increases their capacity to act on issues that they themselves define as important'. The EPF also sees empowerment as a relational concept, in which the patient's environment plays a critical role. Aspects of empowerment include health literacy and a growing recognition of the value of shared decision making and self-management.[3] The EPF has developed a Charter on Patient Empowerment which characterizes an empowered patient. Figure 5.1 summarizes the Charter; more detail is available on the EPF website (www.eu-patient.eu).

1. I am more than my health condition

2. I am empowered to the extent I wish to be

3. I am an equal partner in all decisions related to my health

4. I have the information I need in an easily understandable format, including my own health records

5. My health professionals and our health system actively promote health literacy for all

6. I have the ongoing support I need to manage my own care

7. My experience is a vital measure of healthcare quality

8. I can participate in evaluation and co-designing healthcare services so they work better for everyone

9. Through patient organizations, my voice becomes part of a bigger, united voice

10. Equity and empowerment go hand-in-hand: I want a fair deal for all patients

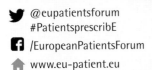

🐦 @eupatientsforum
#PatientsprescribE

f /EuropeanPatientsForum

🏠 www.eu-patient.eu

Figure 5.1 The EPF Charter on Patient Empowerment.

Engagement and empowerment driving high-quality, patient-centred care

The goals of patient engagement and empowerment include improved patient outcomes, i.e. improved quality of life (QOL) and well-being; enhanced adaptation to the long-term effects of treatments; greater independence from healthcare providers and carers; and more effective and sustainable healthcare systems. Important components of patient empowerment and patient engagement include the following:

- Patient participation (otherwise called shared decision making) involves the clinician and patient working collaboratively to select a course of action based on both clinical evidence and the patient's informed preferences.[3] Decision aids providing clear, comprehensible information in an appropriate format will help shared decision making.[4]

- Patient self-management refers to the actions taken by people to recognize, treat and manage their own health.[5]

- Interdisciplinary team work involves different types of staff working together to share expertise and knowledge. Holistic, patient-centred care is emphasized.[6]

- Transition planning to achieve continuity in complex, specialized cancer healthcare is designed to ensure coordination and continuity of care as patients transfer between different locations or levels of care.[7] People want the care they receive to be seamless and to be organized around them and their needs.

Patient engagement and empowerment are ethical imperatives and a rational and evidence-based choice, resulting in better psychosocial and economic health outcomes.[8] Patients experience growing confidence, in general terms and in relation to their expertise and active involvement in their own care and treatment. Venetis et al.[9] found that when patients felt they were listened to, they felt more valued, more positive and more satisfied, and they reported increased confidence and fulfilment. Individuals may experience greater control over their illness, improved treatment outcomes and reduced anxiety; they are thus healthier and enjoy better QOL.[10] Active patients may manage self-care better, thereby easing NHS economic constraints.[11,12]

Some barriers to patient-centred care, patient engagement and patient empowerment remain. For example, some healthcare professionals believe these concepts are not relevant to their practice and dispute their effectiveness in improving outcomes; others aver that individuals with low health literacy may not have the capability that enables them to influence their own care. There is, however, increasing acceptance that in planning cancer services and in the education of healthcare professionals, we should stress the benefits that can flow from active engagement of patients in their care.

Measuring engagement, empowerment and related concepts

Despite growing acceptance of the concept of patient empowerment, uncertainty still exists about how we can measure it. Barr et al.[13] and Eskildsen et al.[14] conducted systematic reviews of scales that measure empowerment. Patient empowerment, patient participation and patient-centredness were examined as general concepts by Castro et al.[15] using a social sciences approach to seek to clarify their meaning. The measurement of empowerment of an individual patient draws on a range of related concepts, the most relevant being self-efficacy (the strength of a person's belief in their ability to succeed in accomplishing a goal, task or challenge);[16] locus of control (how far a person is inclined to see what happens to them as being mostly under the control of external factors or largely under their own control);[17] health orientation, which sets out to measure whether and how far an individual is motivated to engage in healthy behaviours and take responsibility for their own health;[18] and health literacy, which is the extent to which an individual has the capacity to obtain, process and understand health information and services on which they can make appropriate health decisions.[19]

Conclusion

 While some terms will remain imprecisely defined and difficult to measure for some time, a useful distinction may be made between engagement and empowerment. These interrelated concepts and activities are part of an emerging consensus that the partnership between patients and healthcare professionals is essential to achieve the best possible cancer outcomes. The various concepts, definitions, ideas and contributions work together to drive better care (Figure 5.2).

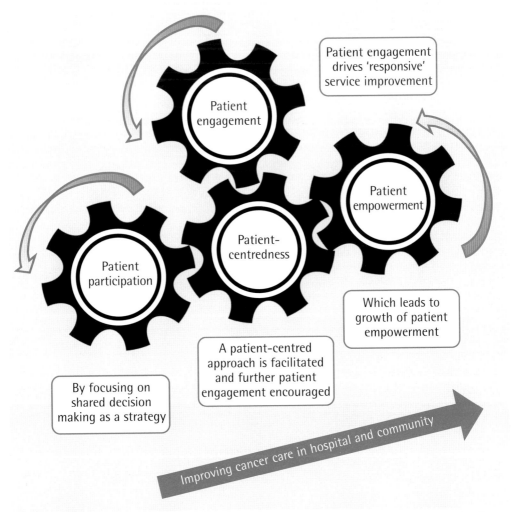

Figure 5.2 Process model showing the concepts of patient participation, engagement, empowerment and patient-centredness in healthcare.

Table 5.1 gives a summary of the tools that can help us improve the quality of care and services, patient experience and patient outcomes. We believe that real benefits can be derived by patients and healthcare professionals from an improved, clearer and shared understanding of engagement and empowerment and their use.

Table 5.1 Engagement and empowerment: practitioner and patient tools.

Exemplars of tools and aids	Further information
The Danish Society for Patient Safety has created a number of initiatives aimed at engaging patients and their families. The *Patient handbook*, for example, is a written guide to hospital care that is designed to facilitate patient engagement. About 10% of all households in Denmark now have a copy of the handbook. The society has adapted the handbook into online question prompts for patients to ask their healthcare professionals, via tablets or cell phones and in paper format	*Patient handbook: a patient's guide to a safer hospital stay*[20]
Motivational interviewing is an empowering technique to facilitate behaviour change by drawing out a patient's own motivations and goals, rather than acceptance of those of the healthcare professional. By placing greater importance on the patient's autonomy, these techniques outperform traditional means of giving advice, in terms of improving health behaviours and adherence to recommendations. The technique is easily adapted for use by non-clinicians, such as local patient and peer support groups	*Motivational interviewing in medical care settings: a systematic review and meta-analysis of randomized controlled trials*[21]
Penny Brohn UK's self-management courses use 'a whole life approach' to help people regain a sense of control over their life following a cancer diagnosis. Attendees report that the promise of regaining control is attractive to them – sometimes over and above a desire to learn more about their condition. One day courses are offered nationwide, and short residential courses are offered too	www.pennybrohn.org.uk
The NHS Expert Patients Programme (EPP) aims to equip people with long-term conditions with the information and skills to better self-manage their health. EPP consists of a series of six weekly sessions, alongside patients with the same condition, facilitated by a tutor. EPP is available for over a dozen chronic conditions, with participants reporting greater confidence and self-control and reduced dependence on healthcare professionals	www.gov.uk/government/case-studies/the-expert-patients-programme
Decision aids internet tools have been developed to help clinicians and carers/patients in their joint decision making about, for example, different adjuvant regimens for early breast cancer; prognosis after neoadjuvant therapy; toxicity; and life expectancy. Such tools use dataset information on thousands of patients, thus allowing much greater accuracy in the decision-making processes	PREDICT (www.predict.nhs.uk) is a well-known decision aid for breast cancer *Internet tools to enhance breast cancer care*[22]

References

1   Funnell MM. Patient empowerment: what does it really mean? *Patient Educ Couns* 2016; 99: 1921–2.

2   Coulter A. Patient engagement – what works? *J Ambulatory Care Manage* 2012; 35: 80–9.

3   Chewning B, Byland B, Shah B, *et al.* Patient preferences for shared decisions: a systematic review. *Patient Educ Couns* 2012; 86: 9–18.

4   Anonymous. An introduction to patient decision aids. *BMJ* 2013; 347: f4147.

5   NHS England (2017). *Supporting self-management/self care.* Available from: www.england.nhs.uk/ourwork/patient-participation/self-care (accessed 3 March 2017).

6   Nancarrow SA, Booth A, Ariss S, *et al.* Ten principles of good interdisciplinary team work. *Hum Resour Health* 2013; 11: 19.

7   Parry C, Mahoney E, Chalmers SA, *et al.* Assessing the quality of transitional care: further applications of the care transitions measure. *Med Care* 2008; 46: 317–22.

8   Editorial. Patient empowerment – who empowers whom? *Lancet* 2012; 379: 1677.

9   Venetis M, Robinson J, Turkiewicz KL, *et al.* An evidence base for patient-centred cancer care: a meta-analysis of studies of observed communication between cancer specialists and their patients. *Patient Educ Couns* 2009; 77: 379–83.

10 Schmidt M, Eckardt R, Scholtz K, *et al.* Patient empowerment improved perioperative quality of care in cancer patients aged ≥65 years – a randomized controlled trial. *PLoS One* 2015; 10: e0137824.

11 Vahedian-Azimi A, Miller AC, Hajiesmaieli M, *et al.* Cardiac rehabilitation using the Family-Centered Empowerment Model versus home-based cardiac rehabilitation in patients with myocardial infarction: a randomised controlled trial. *Open Heart* 2016; 3: e000349.

12 Hibbard JH, Greene J, Overton V. Patients with lower activation associated with higher costs; delivery systems should know their patients' 'scores'. *Health Aff (Millwood)* 2013; 32: 216–22.

13 Barr PJ, Scholl I, Bravo P, *et al.* Assessment of patient empowerment – a systematic review of measures. *PLoS One* 2015; 10: e0126553.

14 Eskildsen NB, Joergensen CR, Thomsen TG, *et al.* Patient empowerment: a systematic review of questionnaires measuring empowerment in cancer patients. *Acta Oncol* 2017; 56: 156–65.

15 Castro E, Van Regenmortel T, Vanhaecht K, *et al.* Patient empowerment, patient participation and patient-centeredness in hospital care: a concept analysis based on a literature review. *Patient Educ Couns* 2016; 99: 1923–39.

16 Lorig K, Chastain RL, Ung E, *et al.* Development and evaluation of a scale to measure perceived self-efficacy in people with arthritis. *Arthritis Rheum* 1989; 32: 37–44.

17 Rotter J. Generalized expectancies for internal versus external control of reinforcement. *Psychol Monogr* 1966; 80: 1–28.

18 DuBenske LL, Burke Beckjord E, Hawkins RP, Gustafson DH. Psychometric evaluation of the Health Information Orientation Scale: a brief measure for assessing health information engagement and apprehension. *J Health Psychol* 2009; 14: 721–30.

19 Dumenci L, Matsuyama R, Riddle DL, *et al.* Measurement of cancer health literacy and identification of patients with limited cancer health literacy. *J Health Commun* 2014; 19 (suppl 2): 205–24.

20 Trygfonden. *Patient handbook: a patient's guide to a safer hospital stay.* Hvidovre: Danish Society for Patient Safety, 2007.

21 Lundahl B, Moleni T, Burke BL, *et al.* Motivational interviewing in medical care settings: a systematic review and meta-analysis of randomized controlled trials. *Patient Educ Couns* 2013; 93: 157–68.

22 Shachar SS, Muss HB. Internet tools to enhance breast cancer care. *NPJ Breast Cancer* 2016; 2: 16011.

06 How Can the GP Support the Patient through the Whole Cancer Journey?

Sinead Clarke, Pete Nightingale, Anthony Cunliffe

Introduction

In the UK we have a unique system of primary care, centred around the GP practice. The GP is often the first port of call for patients and those important to them whenever there is a problem, and general practice aims to provide a service from 'cradle to grave'. The GP and primary care team are therefore in a unique position to support people through a diagnosis of cancer and beyond, enabling them to lead as full a life as possible.

The GP is one member of a multidisciplinary primary care team that is part of a larger community team. The latter includes health and social care professionals such as district nurses and community matrons, community palliative care nurses, mental health workers, social workers, pharmacists and out-of-hours teams.

The term 'patient-centred care' is increasingly being replaced by the term 'person-centred care', which essentially means involving the cancer patient, and taking account of their views, in decisions about their health and care.[1] It looks at their illness and personal goals, treating them as an equal in the process. 'I can plan my care with people who work together to understand me and my carer(s), allow me control, and bring together services to achieve the outcomes important to me.'[2]

Early diagnosis

For many patients, their cancer journey will start in primary care. Some patients' first presentation is to A&E. We know, however, that outcomes for these patients tend to be poorer; so, for most cancers a GP-managed referral route provides the best experience.[3] Providing patient-centred care is imperative for all individuals from the very beginning of their cancer journey. Some may present with an anxiety about cancer, either due to symptoms or, perhaps, as a response to a media campaign or the experience of a friend or relative. Others, however, may present with symptoms that prompt the GP to be suspicious of cancer as a possible diagnosis, without the person having first considered it. Whether it is simply appropriate reassurance that is needed or referral for investigations or via an urgent suspected cancer pathway, clear communication and the provision of all necessary information in the appropriate way are imperative in providing good-quality, truly patient-centred care.

Robust safety netting should be part of any consultation involving a referral to investigate for cancer or to obtain a secondary care opinion. It may come in multiple communication forms including verbal or the provision of appropriate information leaflets, and, like all elements of the consultation, should be tailored to the patient's needs and the level of physician concern. Some patients may present with 'low-risk' symptoms that the GP does not feel need investigating at that time, but that do need to be followed up should they become persistent. Safety netting is just as important for these patients and should involve clear and specific communication.[4]

For patients who have been reassured or whose investigation has been negative, a follow-up consultation provides an opportunity for a 'teachable moment', when a GP could, if felt appropriate, provide information regarding the early signs and symptoms of cancer. Equally important, it provides an excellent opportunity for lifestyle intervention focused around the patient's specific risks.[5]

Living with and beyond cancer

Cancer is increasingly being recognized as a chronic disease. The lifetime risk of developing cancer in the UK is now 50%.[6] Cancer and its treatment often leave people with long-term effects on their mental and/or physical health. Studies by Macmillan Cancer Support have shown the following:[7]

- 90,000 people are affected by gastrointestinal problems including faecal incontinence, diarrhoea and bleeding.
- 350,000 experience sexual difficulties.
- 150,000 have urinary problems.
- 63,000 develop lymphoedema.
- 350,000 have chronic fatigue.
- 240,000 have mental health problems.
- 80,000 have hormonal symptoms.

The recovery package (Figure 6.1) is a series of key interventions which, when delivered together, can greatly improve outcomes for people living with and beyond cancer. In the NHS *Five year forward view*, the recovery package is discussed with details and reference to commissioning guidance on taking the recovery package forward.[8]

The cancer care review is carried out in the GP surgery, normally by a GP or practice nurse, within 6 months of the cancer diagnosis. The aim is to take a holistic look at the patient's needs as she or he comes to the end of active cancer treatment and begins to attempt a return to normal life. This is a challenge in the confines of a 10 min consultation and, although some surgeries allow longer, it is becoming increasingly difficult with the pressures on general practice. A good basis to begin discussions for a cancer care review in general practice is the treatment summary, if there is one.

Treatment summaries are completed by the secondary care team responsible for treating the patient's cancer and include actions for the primary care team relating to such things as ongoing medication or future screening, a summary of the treatment received and follow-up required, possible toxicities or symptoms that require specialist referral, and details of what the patient has been told about the prognosis. A copy is sent to the patient as well as to the GP. Although not universally completed, they are incredibly helpful in enabling good ongoing care and empowerment of the patient, and are detailed in the NHS cancer *Five year forward view*.[8]

There are an estimated 1.5 million cancer carers in the UK and nearly half do not receive any support to care. The report of Macmillan Cancer Support *Under pressure: the growing strain on cancer carers*[9] revealed that up to 70% of cancer carers experience an impact on their mental health, 26% of whom experience depression. GPs can play a key role in supporting cancer carers, as GPs and practice staff are the professionals most likely to identify these carers. All GP surgeries should have carer registers and should signpost to carers' assessments and local sources of support.

The role of the GP in cancer palliative care

Supportive and palliative care has always been a significant and important part of a GP's workload. A major factor in the drive to improve the quality of GP cancer and palliative care was the introduction of the Gold Standards Framework (goldstandardsframework.org.uk) in

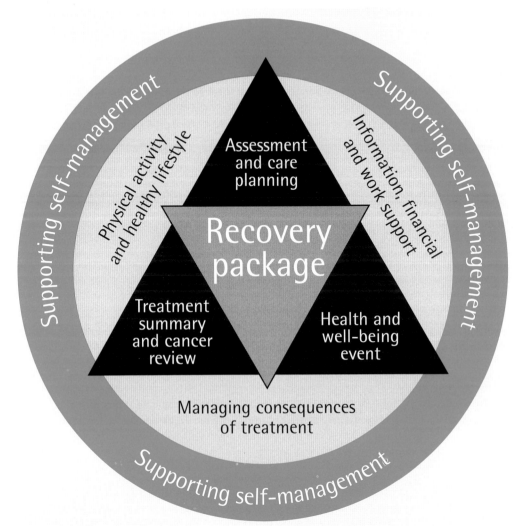

Figure 6.1 The recovery package (reproduced by kind permission of Macmillan Cancer Support).

2000 by Professor Keri Thomas. It became widely used after a national phasing programme supported by the NHS and Macmillan Cancer Support.

Key elements of the Gold Standards Framework, which are also embedded in other quality initiatives,[10] are the need for each patient requiring care to be: (1) identified, (2) assessed, and (3) offered care planning. Primary and secondary care collaboration can greatly assist in these areas.

Identification

Approximately 1% of a GP's patients will die each year.[11] With advances in oncology it is not always clear to GPs when a shift to a more palliative approach to treatment is appropriate.[12] For many, living with cancer has become a chronic disease and they may have limited contact with primary care services. A telephone call from specialist services is welcomed by most GPs if there is disease progression. Letters or emails indicating that a change in the patient's situation has occurred, including what the patient has been told, can be very helpful.

Assessment

GPs providing a high-quality service will have regular, usually monthly, supportive and palliative care meetings. Selecting patients with whom to discuss care in depth is frequently achieved using 'needs-based coding' such as a red, amber, green system. In crude terms, 'red' patients are expected to live days, 'amber' weeks and 'green' months. Specialist advice regarding the expected prognosis and what information patients and their families have been given is usually greatly appreciated.

Planning

Advance care planning is recognized as being important in helping patients achieve their wishes regarding end-of-life care.[13] It has four basic components: (1) what matters to the person, i.e. what gives their life meaning; (2) what they wish to happen; (3) what they do not want to happen; and (4) who will speak for them if they lose mental capacity.

It is helpful for any planning that occurs in secondary care to be shared with the GP to avoid duplication. Do-not-attempt-resuscitation discussions are a good example of this.

In paediatric palliative care, the term 'parallel planning' is often used.[14] It is consistent with a 'hope for the best, plan for the worst' approach. Planning for disease-specific problems such as the risk of treatment-related neutropenia can be integrated with advance care planning to produce a personalized care plan. Plans may then be shared electronically if appropriate.[15]

Conclusion

General practice and community teams are extremely important in supporting cancer patients and those important to them throughout the cancer journey. The closer primary and secondary care teams can work together, the more likely we are to be able to achieve true patient-/person-centred care for all.

References

1 Royal College of General Practitioners (2014). *Inquiry into patient centred care in the 21st century: implications for general practice and primary care.* Available from: www.rcgp.org.uk/policy/rcgp-policy-areas/inquiry-into-patient-centred-care-in-the-21st-century.aspx (accessed 5 April 2017).

2 National Voices (2013). *A narrative for person-centred coordinated care.* NHS England publication gateway reference number 00076. Available from: www.nationalvoices.org.uk/publications/our-publications/narrative-person-centred-coordinated-care (accessed 5 April 2017).

3 Zhou Y, Abel GA, Hamilton W, *et al.* Diagnosis of cancer as an emergency: a critical review of current evidence. *Nat Rev Clin Oncol* 2017; 14: 45–56.

4 Nicholson BD, Mant D, Bankhead C. Can safety-netting improve cancer detection in patients with vague symptoms? *BMJ* 2016; 355: i5515.

5 Renzi C, Whitaker KL, Winstanley K, *et al.* Unintended consequences of an 'all-clear' diagnosis for potential cancer symptoms: a nested qualitative interview study with primary care patients. *Br J Gen Pract* 2016; 66: e158–70.

6   Ahmad AS, Ormiston-Smith N, Sasieni PD. Trends in the lifetime risk of developing cancer in Great Britain: comparison of risk for those born from 1930 to 1960. *Br J Cancer* 2015: 112: 943–7.

7   Royal College of General Practitioners, Macmillan Cancer Support (2013). *Consequences of cancer and treatment*. Available from: www.rcgp.org.uk/coc (accessed 5 April 2017).

8   NHS England (2016). *Achieving world-class cancer outcomes: taking the strategy forward. Five year forward view.* NHS England publication gateway reference number 05215. Available from: www.england.nhs.uk/wp-content/uploads/2016/05/cancer-strategy.pdf (accessed 1 May 2017).

9   Macmillan Cancer Support (2016). *Under pressure: the growing strain on cancer carers.* Available from: www.macmillan.org.uk/documents/campaigns/under-pressure-the-growing-strain-on-cancer-carers-macmillan-cancer-support-september-2016.pdf (accessed 5 April 2017).

10 NHS Cheshire and Merseyside Strategic Clinical Networks (2015). *Advance care planning framework.* Available from: www.nwcscnsenate.nhs.uk/files/6514/4284/8049/Advance_Care_Planning_Framework_2015-18_FINAL.pdf?PDFPATHWAY=PDF (accessed 5 April 2017).

11 Dying Matters. Available from: www.dyingmatters.org/gp (accessed 5 April 2017).

12 Murray SA, Boyd K, Sheikh A. Palliative care in chronic illnesses. We need to move from prognostic paralysis to active total care. *BMJ* 2005; 330: 611–12.

13 Mullick A, Martin J, Sallnow L. An introduction to advance care planning in practice. *BMJ* 2013; 347: f6064.

14 British Association of Perinatal Medicine (2010). *Palliative care (supportive and end of life care). A framework for clinical practice in perinatal medicine.* Available from: http://bapm.org/publications/documents/guidelines/Palliative_Care_Report_final_%20Aug10.pdf (accessed 5 April 2017).

15 Petrova M, Riley J, Abel J, Barclay S. Crash course in EPaCCS (Electronic Palliative Care Coordination Systems): 8 years of successes and failures in patient data sharing to learn from. *BMJ Support Palliat Care* doi: 10.1136/bmjspcare-2015-001059.

07 Making a Difference: the True Value of Voluntary Sector and NHS Collaboration for Cancer Patients, Carers and Families

Laura Lee

Introduction

Today, more people are living longer with – and surviving – cancer than ever before. Better treatment and better understanding of the disease are helping to improve the quality of life of people living with cancer, and so a phrase that has always been at the heart of what we do at Maggie's (www.maggiescentres.órg) 'living well with cancer' has become a possibility for more and more people. At the same time, longer life expectancy generally means more people are expected to have cancer at some point in their life. In the UK there are currently 2 million people living with or after cancer; this figure is steadily rising, with more than 300,000 new diagnoses each year.[1] In other words, it is estimated that half of us will have cancer at some point in our lifetime.[1]

The rising number of those living with a cancer diagnosis means that people are experiencing new, long-term psychological and physical consequences as a result of cancer and its treatment. As the number continues to rise, so the demand for support and care increases, putting pressure on limited NHS resources. The rising demand means that collaboration with the voluntary sector and recognition of the role it can play has never been more vital for the future of cancer care.

Shared values

The voluntary sector and the NHS have shared values: we both want the best for people with cancer and their families. But we are not always good at recognizing what else outside cancer treatment may be helpful in supporting people fully. We agree that management of care should be proactive, holistic, preventive and person-focused. But, as most people working in the NHS and voluntary sector would acknowledge, there is still some way to go to reach a truly coordinated approach to treatment, support and care.

There are many voluntary and community organizations providing health and care services in the UK, and the NHS is increasingly looking to them for long-term partnerships rather than 'quick fix' solutions. Instead of simply helping people once they are ill, the mission must be to support people to live well, to prevent ill health where possible, and to reach the most vulnerable people in society. In order to achieve this, the NHS needs to acknowledge its own limitations and share them with the voluntary sector. There are, however, many barriers to overcome before this can happen effectively. The biggest of these is that the NHS is such a vast and complex organization that it can be difficult to get a foothold on sharing issues effectively. With hospitals and practices all over the country, initiating a high level of change is a huge challenge.

Working together

The essence of the NHS *Five year forward view*, a plan published in 2014 by NHS England, is to seek 'a new relationship with patients and communities'.[2] How can we work together to achieve this? How can organizations in the voluntary sector, like Maggie's, help people to get the best out of their treatment on the NHS? And how can we work together to make sure people feel like active participants in their own treatment? One simple step would be to help people become more involved in decisions about their care. At Maggie's we approach everyone who visits our centres by asking 'What matters to you?', rather than 'What's the matter with you?', in order to find out what is important to the individual and their loved ones. The NHS is not currently able to adequately offer people this kind of service. Its primary function is to provide the best possible medical care, and the amazing doctors and nurses who work for the NHS simply do not have the time to answer all of the overwhelming questions that come with a cancer diagnosis, such as 'What does this mean?', 'How do I tell my family?' and 'What do I do now?'

People tell us that what they want and need from the voluntary sector is time and space to deal with their individual needs and concerns, and to have support with the non-clinical elements of having cancer, such as eating well, managing anxiety and stress, coping with relationships and family, and understanding benefits and financial aspects. We in the voluntary sector have our own hurdles to overcome. We sometimes do not collaborate well, either with the NHS or with other organizations. This is possibly because we operate in a very competitive market for funding and donations; but we can also find ourselves criticizing each other and the NHS, the very organization we should be trying to help. The voluntary sector can also be set in its ways, and so it is also important that we are willing and able to adapt to the changing nature of healthcare.

In many ways, Maggie's developed from a desire to be what the NHS is not. Maggie's Centres are designed to be the antithesis of an NHS hospital (Figure 7.1). They are beautiful buildings,

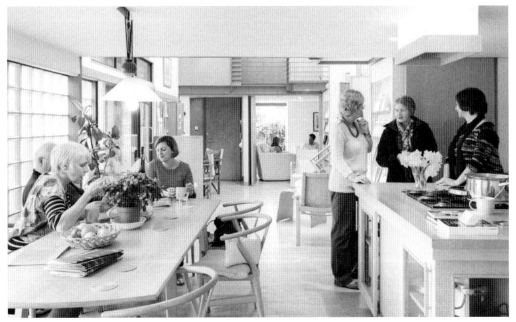

Figure 7.1 Inside Maggie's Edinburgh, the first Maggie's Centre, which opened in 1996 (photograph by Philip Durrant).

carefully designed so that people will want to spend time in them. Visitors are welcome without an appointment and can stay as long as they want during opening hours. When they come to Maggie's, visitors choose what to do and where to go, which elements of our programme of support they would like to get involved in, or whether they would prefer just to make themselves a cup of tea and sit looking out of the window. There is no time limit on the support we offer. People can continue to visit Maggie's for as long as they like, even after their cancer has gone. Indeed, people are equally welcome at Maggie's whether they have, or have had, cancer themselves, or know someone who has. Maggie's does not provide medical treatment, but we are on hand to give information and offer a programme of support that can improve the well-being of people with cancer. Rather than polarizing, these differences are precisely what make Maggie's and the NHS such a good fit. Every one of our 20 UK centres is in the grounds of a major NHS cancer hospital and is there at the invitation of the local trust. Our programme of support is developed with the input of leading clinicians to complement medical treatment; 42% of all people who come to Maggie's are directed to us by hospital staff. We are here to help people at all stages of their cancer experience, as well as their family and friends, whatever their age or economic background.

When Maggie's goes to a new hospital to begin discussions about building a new centre we always try to overlook our own agenda and understand each community's and their local NHS body's needs. One common need is time. We know how stretched the time of those working in the NHS is, which is why we help their patients with simple things like understanding the information they have been given by medical staff, and speaking to their families and loved ones about their diagnosis.

We recognize that there can be a perception, within the NHS and among the public, that the voluntary sector is amateur and led by volunteers – a nice place to go or be. There is also an idea that, unlike the NHS, charities do not have to demonstrate the impact their work has. Today, however, more and more organizations like Maggie's are delivering a professionally led, evidence-based level of care and support, which we know has a positive impact and makes a significant difference to people living with cancer.

Being a charity gives us the freedom to be flexible and creative in our care for people with cancer and their families, friends and carers in a way that the NHS cannot. This is why we strive to share our spaces with our colleagues in the NHS, encouraging them to hold their own support groups in our centres, or even for staff to come and have their lunch in our gardens so that they can experience at first hand what Maggie's offers, and so that we can emphasize that we are working together rather than in competition. The voluntary sector can be a place for the NHS to try out or pilot new kinds of treatment and therapies that it may be looking at adopting.

I believe we can change the way the NHS and voluntary sector work together. We can offer more support to those who need it if we show each other more understanding and respect each other's work and knowledge in our respective fields. It is important that we continue to learn from each other and build on our strengths so that together we can improve the quality of life for everyone affected by cancer.

References

1 Cancer Research UK. *Cancer statistics for the UK*. Available from: www.cancerresearchuk.org/health-professional/cancer-statistics (accessed 8 May 2017).

2 NHS England (2014). *Five year forward view*. Available from: www.england.nhs.uk/wp-content/uploads/2014/10/5yfv-web.pdf (accessed 8 May 2017).

08 Cancer Survivorship

Lynn Calman, Claire Foster

Background

Improvements in cancer survival have been marked over the last 40 years due to screening, earlier diagnosis and improvements in and access to treatment. It is predicted that half of people diagnosed with cancer in England and Wales in 2010–2011 will survive for at least 10 years.[1] This rate has doubled since the 1970s.[1] The current UK 10 year survival rates are around 80% for breast cancer and 84% for prostate cancer.[2]

Cancer is still a leading cause of morbidity and mortality. In England and Wales 40% of all preventable deaths are caused by cancer.[3] The poor survival in some cancers has changed little since the 1970s. For example, lung cancer survival remains very poor, with only 10% of patients surviving 5 years and 5% surviving 10 years.[1] More than a quarter of all people with lung cancer die within a year of diagnosis.[4] It has been estimated that 2.5 million people were living with and beyond cancer in the UK in 2015 and this number is set to increase to an estimated 4 million by 2030.[5]

In response to the growing number of people surviving cancer there has been increasing focus over the last few decades on the quality of survival as well as on the number of disease-free years. Survivorship has various definitions and can include anyone diagnosed with cancer, from diagnosis to end of life.[6]

Impact of cancer and its treatment on everyday life

Cancer and its treatment can have a considerable and long-term impact on everyday life.[7-9] Cancer survivors may face a range of challenges including physical problems, poorer quality of life (QOL), psychological distress, sexual problems, problems with social relationships and financial concerns.[9] An estimated 625,000 cancer survivors in the UK are facing poor health or disability.[10] At least 350,000 are living with chronic fatigue, 240,000 with mental health problems, 200,000 with severe pain after curative treatment, 150,000 with urinary problems such as incontinence and 90,000 with gastrointestinal problems, including faecal incontinence, diarrhoea and bleeding.[10] Some consequences may emerge 5 or 10 years after treatment (late effects) and can have a significant impact. For example, some chemotherapy can increase the risk of heart disease, and long-term hormone therapy is related to osteoporosis.[10]

Important elements of survivorship

Cancer survivorship is broader than length of survival or detection of recurrence and symptoms. It includes psychosocial aspects such as coping with disruption to one's life, confidence to manage consequences of treatment, living with uncertainty, lifestyle changes and so on.[11] It can also include disruption to one's social role and identity.[12] Foster and Fenlon's conceptual model of recovery of health and well-being following cancer treatment attempts to draw these elements together from empirical research findings (Figure 8.1).[13] They hypothesize that health and well-being in survivorship are positively associated with support for the individual (e.g. from health and social care, community, family and friends), other personal attributes (e.g. resilience, health beliefs), the

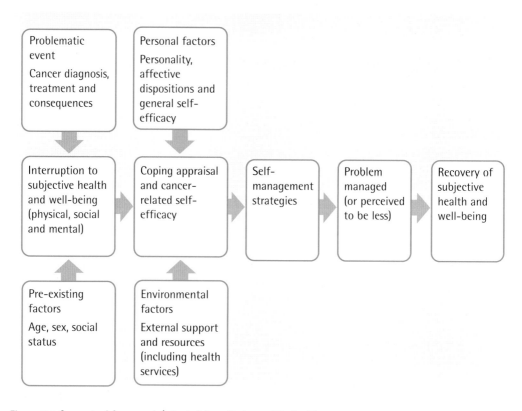

Figure 8.1 Conceptual framework (adapted from Foster and Fenlon[13]).

patient's confidence (e.g. self-efficacy), and self-management strategies used to manage problems faced as a consequence of the cancer and its treatment.[13]

Cancer as a long-term condition

As a consequence of rising survival rates, more people are experiencing cancer, not as a life-limiting 'incurable' disease, but as a life-changing and chronic rather than an acute condition. As such it involves not cure, but work to identify and prevent recurrence, change lifestyle, and manage exacerbations, complexity and uncertainty. Increasingly patients are held accountable for this work.[14] This results in significant challenges to healthcare and how the interactions between services and contexts in the hospital and community are managed. There is growing recognition that healthcare services need to adapt to better support people living with and beyond cancer.

Increased understanding about the 2.5 million cancer survivors in the UK is helping to explain the differences in 'complexity, intensity and longevity' of need and the impact of factors such as age, sex, multiple morbidity and deprivation on outcomes.[15] For example, the number of people aged 65 and over living with cancer has grown by 25% in the 5 years to 2015.[5] Owing to an ageing population, living with comorbidities alongside cancer is common, bringing additional complexity and potential burden. The number of people with comorbidities is set to increase in England from 1.9 million in 2008 to 2.9 million by 2018.[16] Although the evidence for managing the care of patients with multimorbidity is limited,[17] an approach to disease management that focuses on multimorbidity may be needed to address patients' needs adequately.[16]

Health service innovation

Patients have highlighted the need for support to manage the impact of cancer on everyday life.[7] Most of the time, people living with cancer, together with those close to them, manage their own health and well-being at home without the input of health professionals. People can be unprepared for the impact cancer and its treatment can have on their life: they may feel vulnerable and experience a loss of confidence, and may struggle to access care and support.[9,13,18,19] In light of the view that cancer can be managed as a chronic illness,[20] it has been recognized that patients could benefit from access to a model of care similar to that used in long-term conditions incorporating supported self-management.[21] Self-management support for long-term conditions is embedded in UK health policy and there is increasing evidence that supporting people to manage their own heath has positive outcomes including improved QOL and reduced use of health services.[22]

There has been a call to redesign healthcare using the principle of what has been described as minimally disruptive medicine.[23] This is complex whole-systems change, which aims to put the patient at the centre of healthcare.[14] Initiatives to support cancer survivors across the globe have driven a significant rise in research and service development in this area. The UK National Cancer Survivorship Initiative (NCSI) was established to understand the needs of those living with cancer and develop models of care that meet their needs. In 2013, the NCSI published *Living with and beyond cancer: taking action to improve outcomes* to support commissioners, providers and others to improve cancer survivorship outcomes and suggested interventions that could support the population.[6] Following on from the NCSI, the living with and beyond cancer programme established in 2014 is focusing on tackling the recommendations and priorities identified by the NCSI.[24]

Supporting survivors to manage the consequences of cancer and its treatment

Self-management support is multifaceted.[25] For people with long-term conditions it has been defined as being an active partner in determining outcomes that are important and how to achieve them; working in collaboration with healthcare providers; being supported to build knowledge, skills, confidence and resilience to manage the impact of symptoms and limitations in order to live a full and meaningful life; and being enabled to access support within and beyond health services to better manage health and well-being.[22]

For cancer survivors, self-management includes managing the consequences of cancer and its treatment, such as symptoms; seeking support when appropriate; recognizing and reporting signs and symptoms of possible disease progression; and making lifestyle changes to promote health, well-being and survival.[26] People need varying degrees of support from healthcare professionals and others to achieve this.

Tailoring aftercare according to need

In light of the increasing number of survivors and growing evidence of their needs, it has become clear that some patents do well after cancer treatment and some experience problems and poor recovery. There is a growing view that personalized or tailored care is important, as current models of aftercare are not meeting patients' needs.[27] One way of achieving this is through risk-stratified care, which has been a central focus of UK survivorship programmes.[6,24] Although risk stratification is considered as having potential to deliver personalized care and improve consistency across cancer centres, it has a weak evidence base in cancer survivorship.[28] In particular there is a paucity of tools for stratifying individual risk, including which patients are at risk of which adverse outcomes, the magnitude of the risk, the significance of the impact of outcomes for the individual and the availability of evidence-based interventions.[28]

Patients have access to a holistic needs assessment and cancer care review (to assess current need), but we are still some way from finding optimal methods of assessment for risk stratification to identify patients who are most at risk of poor recovery, so that the appropriate level of intervention can be offered.[28] At present the methods used to determine what type of support people receive after treatment is driven by clinical characteristics such as risk of recurrence.[28] The role of psychosocial factors in risk stratification has received less attention. Data are emerging to indicate that psychosocial factors such as confidence to manage illness-related problems (e.g. self-efficacy) are important predictors of recovery experience.[29]

Conclusion

The number of people receiving a cancer diagnosis is set to rise. Many will be living with disruption due to physical, psychological, social, vocational and other consequences of their disease and/or its treatment. The role of healthcare will be to support those living with and beyond a diagnosis of cancer to enable them to live as fulfilling a life as possible in the short, medium and longer term. Assessing level of need and risk is important not only early in the patient's pathway but during and after treatment and regularly over time. This will allow services to be targeted or tailored according to need and risk, rather than follow the one-size-fits-all approach which the system is struggling to deliver and which is not currently meeting patients' needs.

References

1 Cancer Research UK (2017). *Cancer survival statistics.* Available from: www.cancerresearchuk.org/health-professional/cancer-statistics/survival (accessed April 2017).

2 Cancer Research UK (2017). *Cancer statistics for the UK.* Available from: www.cancerresearchuk.org/health-professional/cancer-statistics (accessed 9 June 2017).

3 Office for National Statistics (2017). *Avoidable mortality in England and Wales: 2014.* Available from: www.ons.gov.uk/peoplepopulationandcommunity/healthandsocialcare/causesofdeath/bulletins/avoidablemortalityinenglandandwales/2014#main-points (accessed April 2017).

4 Maddams J, Utley M, Møller H. A person–time analysis of hospital activity among cancer survivors in England. *Br J Cancer* 2011; 105 (suppl 1): S38–45.

5 Maddams J, Utley M, Møller H. Projections of cancer prevalence in the United Kingdom, 2010–2040. *Br J Cancer* 2012; 107: 1195–202.

6 Department of Health, Macmillan Cancer Support, NHS Improvement. *Living with and beyond cancer: taking action to improve outcomes.* London: Department of Health, 2013.

7 Corner J, Wright D, Hopkinson J, *et al.* The research priorities of patients attending UK cancer treatment centres: findings from a modified nominal group study. *Br J Cancer* 2007; 96: 875–81.

8 Hewitt M, Rowland JH, Yancik R. Cancer survivors in the United States: age, health, and disability. *J Gerontol A Biol Sci Med Sci* 2003; 58: 82–91.

9 Foster C, Haviland J, Winter J, *et al.* Pre-surgery depression and confidence to manage problems predict recovery trajectories of health and wellbeing in the first two years following colorectal cancer: results from the CREW cohort study. *PLoS One* 2016; 11: e0155434.

10 Macmillan Cancer Support (2013). *Throwing light on the consequences of cancer and its treatment.* Available from: www.macmillan.org.uk/documents/aboutus/research/researchandevaluationreports/throwinglightontheconsequencesofcanceranditstreatment.pdf (accessed August 2016).

11 Lent RW. Restoring emotional well-being: a theoretical model. In: Feuerstein M, ed. *Handbook of cancer survivorship.* New York: Springer, 2007; 231–48.

12 Bury M. Chronic illness as biographical disruption. *Sociol Health Illn* 1982; 4: 167–82.

13 Foster C, Fenlon D. Recovery and self-management support following primary cancer treatment. *Br J Cancer* 2011; 105 (suppl 1): S21–8.

14 May C, Eton D, Boehmer K, *et al.* Rethinking the patient: using burden of treatment theory to understand the changing dynamics of illness. *BMC Health Serv Res* 2014; 14: 281.

15 McConnell H, White R, Maher J, Macmillan Cancer Support (2017). *Three cancer groups. Explaining the different complexity, intensity and longevity of broad clinical needs.* Available from: www.macmillan.org.uk/_images/three-cancer-groups_tcm9-297577.pdf (accessed April 2017).

16 Department of Health (2014). *Comorbidities: a framework of principles for system-wide action.* Available from: www.gov.uk/government/publications/better-care-for-people-with-2-or-more-long-term-conditions (accessed August 2016).

17 Smith SM, Soubhi H, Fortin M, *et al.* Managing patients with multimorbidity: systematic review of interventions in primary care and community settings *BMJ* 2012; 345: e5205.

18 Jefford M, Karahalios E, Pollard A, *et al.* Survivorship issues following treatment completion – results from focus groups with Australian cancer survivors and health professionals. *J Cancer Surviv* 2008; 2: 20–32.

19 Hewitt M, Greenfield S, Stovall E. *From cancer patient to cancer survivor: lost in transition.* Washington, DC: National Academies Press, 2005.

20 McCorkle R, Ercolano E, Lazenby M, *et al.* Self-management: enabling and empowering patients living with cancer as a chronic illness. *CA Cancer J Clin* 2011; 61: 50–62.

21 McConnell H, White R, Maher J (2017). Understanding variations. Outcomes for people diagnosed with cancer and implications for service provision. Available from: www.macmillan.org.uk/_images/understanding-variations_tcm9-298045.pdf (accessed April 2017).

22 The Health Foundation. *A practical guide to self-management support. Key components for successful implementation.* London: The Health Foundation, 2015.

23 May C, Montori VM, Mair FS. We need minimally disruptive medicine. *BMJ* 2009; 339: b2803.

24 NHS England (2017). *Living with and beyond cancer.* Available from: www.england.nhs.uk/cancer/living/ (accessed April 2017).

25 Johnston B, Rogerson L, Macijauskiene J, *et al.* An exploration of self-management support in the context of palliative nursing: a modified concept analysis. *BMC Nurs* 2014; 13: 21.

26 Foster C. Survivorship and self-management in cancer care. In: Wyatt D, Hubert-Williams N, eds. *Cancer and cancer care.* London: Sage, 2015.

27 Santin O, Mills M, Treanor C, Donnelly MA. A comparative analysis of the health and well-being of cancer survivors to the general population. *Support Care Cancer* 2012; 20: 2545–52.

28 Watson EK, Rose PW, Neal RD, *et al.* Personalised cancer follow-up: risk stratification, needs assessment or both? *Br J Cancer* 2012; 106: 1–5.

29 Foster C, Wright D, Hill H, *et al.* Psychosocial implications of living 5 years or more following a cancer diagnosis: a systematic review of the research evidence. *Eur J Cancer Care (Engl)* 2009; 18: 223–47.

09 Survivorship and Rehabilitation: Recommendations from a European Perspective

Tit Albreht, Christine Berling, Claudia Ferrari, Stein Kaasa, Luzia Travado

Introduction

The substantially increasing number of cancer survivors in Europe led the EU Joint Action on Cancer Control (CanCon) to focus on survivorship and rehabilitation as part of the *European guide on quality improvement in comprehensive cancer control.*[1] The objective was to take into account the psychosocial needs of patients and improve quality of life (QOL) for cancer patients through support, rehabilitation and palliative care.[2] A patient-centred approach is of paramount importance in planning care provision for cancer survivors and ensuring optimal QOL. The quality of care for cancer survivors is impaired if there is poor coordination, if communication is lacking, or if there is uncertainty about the key contact person in follow-up. This can result in poorer psychosocial outcomes and unmet needs. The report identified the importance of the advice from the US Institute of Medicine that specific templates should be developed for the follow-up of cancer survivors and used in the development of survivorship care plans to overcome the many factors impeding good QOL for cancer survivors.[3] It is clear, however, that such care plans are still used to only a modest degree because of the difficulty of integrating them into practice and the resources required to do so. The improvements in cancer survival that we are observing reflect in part the increasing scale and quality of clinical cancer research and trials. The European Organisation for Research and Treatment of Cancer has responded to this challenge by highlighting the importance of survivorship and addressing this need through research and innovation.[4]

Key areas for recommendations

The main messages of the EU CanCon initiative for survivorship and rehabilitation are shown in Table 9.1. In describing cancer survivorship, CanCon drew on the definition provided by the US National Coalition for Cancer Survivorship (www.canceradvocacy.org) which describes it as 'the experience of living with, through and beyond a diagnosis of cancer'. This inclusive definition means that a cancer survivor is anyone who has had a diagnosis of cancer and who is still alive. This includes individuals receiving treatment with curative, life-prolonging or palliative intent, as well as those in follow-up.[3,5,6] The best approaches employ survivorship care plans that cover both medical and non-medical aspects of care. Models reported include the shared care model and the availability of specialized survivorship clinics,[7] as well as collaboration between primary and hospital care. Care plans need to establish how responsibility should be shared. Evidence suggests that there is considerable added value for patients and healthcare systems with the use of survivorship care plans even though they are currently far from routine.

The CanCon group drew on recommendations from the Institute of Medicine[3] and the National Cancer Survivorship Initiative[8] and also reviewed results from other countries. Six key areas were identified.

Table 9.1 Survivorship and rehabilitation: main messages from the CanCon project.[1]

- Cancer survivors' follow-up, late effects management and tertiary prevention needs should be anticipated, personalized and implemented into care pathways, with active participation of survivors and relatives

- Improvement is needed in early detection of patients' needs, and their access to rehabilitation, psychosocial and palliative care services is required

- An integrated and multi-professional care approach is required with coordination of community care providers and services to implement a survivorship care plan that enhances patient self-management and QOL

- For child, adolescent and young adult survivors, late health and psychosocial effects of cancer and its treatments should be anticipated and addressed

- More research in the area of survivorship is needed to provide data on late effects, as well as the impact and cost-effectiveness of supportive care, rehabilitation, and palliative and psychosocial care interventions

- Medical follow-up: management of late effects, and tertiary prevention.
- Palliative care in primary and secondary care.
- Psychological support.
- Social rehabilitation including employment issues.
- Empowerment of cancer survivors.
- Multidisciplinary approach and coordination of care providers.

In addition there were four cross-cutting themes.
- Care for childhood cancer survivors.
- Inequalities in survivorship.
- Cancer information and data registration.
- Research.

Literature review: themes and key areas

The themes and key areas were subjected to a literature review and a critical appraisal, and the results were incorporated into the recommendations. A total of 151 publications were identified. The definition of a survivorship plan by the US National Cancer Institute was found to be useful: 'A detailed plan for a patient's follow-up care after treatment for a disease ends.'[9] In cancer, the plan is based on the type of cancer and the treatment the patient has received. A survivorship care plan may include schedules for physical examinations and medical tests. Follow-up care also monitors health problems that may occur months or years after treatment ends; it may also include information to help meet the emotional, social, legal and financial needs of the patient. It may include referrals to specialists, and recommendations for a healthy lifestyle, such as changes in diet and exercise and stopping smoking. The findings are summarized below.

Medical follow-up and management of late effects

Survivorship care plans have to take account of the need to assess the direct and indirect effects of cancer and its treatment, such as specific organ toxicity, fatigue, pain, depression, anxiety, sleep disturbances, and sexual or fertility problems. Patients need to be asked directly by systematic collection of patient-reported outcome measures. Social issues may be very pressing for cancer patients, including the impact of reduced income or loss of employment. Many of these issues are particularly important, and still incompletely understood, for children, adolescents and young adults surviving cancer. Survivorship care plans identify and facilitate patients' rehabilitation needs.

Tertiary prevention

Follow-up and active management of survivorship should promote a healthy lifestyle, physical activity, and the avoidance of risk factors for further cancers, such as sun exposure, alcohol consumption and smoking.

Patients with advanced cancer

Symptom control and the integration of supportive and palliative care into cancer care have been shown to be beneficial in this group. This approach is becoming increasingly important as more patients are living longer on tumour-directed treatment. Many of these patients are suffering from physical and psychological symptoms and distress.

A patient-centred approach to long-term follow-up

The needs of cancer survivors are complex and multidimensional. They include psychological support and social rehabilitation, supportive and palliative care, and management of the medical aspects of their illness. A patient-centred approach involves patients in taking decisions about the approach to their survivorship care and takes account of the impact of care packages on health-related QOL (HRQOL). Psychological factors include fear of recurrence, fatigue, sexual difficulties and emotional changes (e.g. anxiety and depression), all of which have negative influences on QOL. Psychological interventions can reduce psychological morbidities and improve patients' QOL; access to these is an important part of survivorship care. The CanCon initiative drew attention to the importance of evidence-based palliative, supportive and psychosocial care in clinical practice. Considerable emphasis has been placed on support in returning to work, the positive effects of early psychosocial interventions, and the role of legislation to protect employment for cancer patients. CanCon emphasized the importance of integrated, multidisciplinary care, patient empowerment and the self-management perspective for cancer survivors (see Chapters 5, 7 and 13).

An integrated survivorship and rehabilitation care model is shown in Figure 9.1. It emphasizes a multidisciplinary, patient-centred approach to survivorship care. Key aspects include clarity around an early and personalized follow-up programme agreed with each cancer survivor; the use of adequate and updated information and long-term effects provided to cancer survivors; the integration of tertiary prevention into the plan; and a patient-centred approach to the provision of care, including psychological and social support and a focus on maintaining HRQOL. A wide range of health professionals need to be involved in the implementation of effective management for cancer survivors, both in the hospital and the community.

There remains a great deal to learn about optimal survivorship care. Clinical research is needed to evaluate optimal care plans using outcome measures including patient-reported QOL. Modern informatics and communications technology will help link patients to their appropriate professional carers in both the hospital and community and may make it easier to provide comprehensive care for cancer survivors and ensure the best QOL for them in the long term.

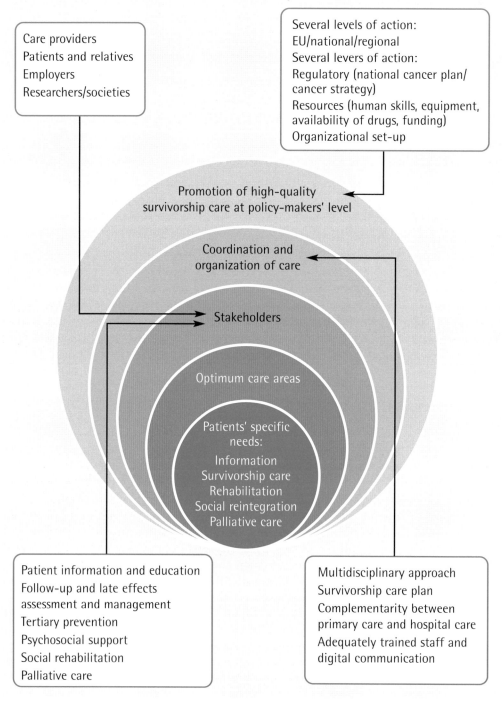

Care providers
Patients and relatives
Employers
Researchers/societies

Several levels of action:
EU/national/regional
Several levers of action:
Regulatory (national cancer plan/
cancer strategy)
Resources (human skills, equipment,
availability of drugs, funding)
Organizational set-up

Promotion of high-quality
survivorship care at policy-makers' level

Coordination and
organization of care

Stakeholders

Optimum care areas

Patients' specific
needs:
Information
Survivorship care
Rehabilitation
Social reintegration
Palliative care

Patient information and education
Follow-up and late effects
assessment and management
Tertiary prevention
Psychosocial support
Social rehabilitation
Palliative care

Multidisciplinary approach
Survivorship care plan
Complementarity between
primary care and hospital care
Adequately trained staff and
digital communication

Figure 9.1 Integrated survivorship and rehabilitation care model showing the different components of an effective European organizational survivorship care model using an integrated and personalized approach (adapted from Albreht et al.[1]).

References

1 Albreht T, Borrás Andrés JM, Dalmas M, *et al.* Survivorship and rehabilitation: policy recommendations for quality improvement in cancer survivorship and rehabilitation in EU member states. In: Albreht T, Kiasuwa R, Van den Bulcke M, eds. *European guide on quality improvement in comprehensive cancer control.* Ljubljana: National Institute of Public Health, 2017; 135–64.

2 Council of the European Union (2008). *Council conclusions on reducing the burden of cancer.* Available from: www.eu2008.si/en/News_and_Documents/Council_Conclusions/June/0609_EPSCO-cancer.pdf (accessed 25 March 2017).

3 Hewitt M, Greenfield S, Stovall E, eds. *From cancer patient to cancer survivor: lost in transition.* Washington, DC: National Academies Press, 2006.

4 Liu L, O'Donnell P, Sullivan R, *et al.* Cancer in Europe: death sentence or life sentence? *Eur J Cancer* 2016; 65: 150–5.

5 Wolff SN. The burden of cancer survivorship. A pandemic of treatment success. In: Feuerstein M, ed. *Handbook of cancer survivorship.* New York: Springer, 2006; 7–18.

6 Keesing S, McNamara B, Rosenwax L. Cancer survivors' experience of using survivorship care plans: a systematic review of qualitative studies. *J Cancer Surviv* 2015; 9: 260–8.

7 Earle CC. Quality of care. In: Feuerstein M, ed. *Handbook of cancer survivorship.* New York: Springer, 2006; 19–42.

8 Department of Health, Macmillan Cancer Support, NHS Improvement (2010). *The National Cancer Survivorship Initiative vision.* Available from: https://annawallacecouk.files.wordpress.com/2011/11/ncsi-vision-document.pdf (accessed 12 July 2017).

9 National Cancer Institute (2010). *Follow-up care after cancer treatment.* Available from: www.cancer.gov/about-cancer/coping/survivorship/follow-up-care/follow-up-fact-sheet (accessed 24 April 2017).

10 Improving Quality of Life after Cancer Treatment

Jane Maher, Lesley Smith, Louisa Petchey

Background

The importance of the challenge facing the growing number of long-term cancer survivors has been highlighted in previous chapters on cancer survivorship and survivorship and rehabilitation in the EU. In 2010 the National Cancer Survivorship Initiative (NCSI) confirmed that a significant minority of cancer survivors had unmet needs after treatment, and identified three questions.[1]

- What are the potential consequences of cancer and its treatment?
- How prevalent are they?
- What can be done to prevent or reduce their impact on quality of life (QOL)?

In this chapter we review the clinical approaches available for managing these consequences and highlight some clinically challenging examples. At least one in four cancer survivors (approximately 625,000 people in the UK) have one or more physical or psychological difficulties as a result of their cancer or treatment which have a long-term effect on their lives, including 350,000 with severe fatigue, 200,000 with moderate to severe pain, 150,000 with urinary problems and 90,000 with faecal urgency, incontinence, diarrhoea, etc.[2]

People living with the consequences of cancer treatment

People with (or at risk of) the consequences of cancer treatment can be placed into three broad groups which differ in terms of the severity and prevalence of the consequences with which they live. Categorization into groups helps define optimal approaches to the identification and management of people's care needs.

Group 1: Severe, chronic consequences requiring specialist support

These consequences stand out as having the highest impact and often the highest profile among the consequences of cancer treatment.

- They affect a small number of people (1–5% of those treated).
- They have a severe impact on QOL over many years.
- They often affect multiple organs/body areas, and therefore require input from multiple clinical specialities.

Example: Radiation-induced brachial plexopathy

A radiotherapy technique to treat breast cancer, most commonly used in the 1970s, led to complex regional pain, loss of arm movement, and tissue damage. Patients were identified through a national call, and published guidance was prioritized. Multidisciplinary assessment was found to be essential to diagnose this condition and to determine the most appropriate level of care, including specialist rehabilitation to reduce distress and delay disability.[3] This led to specialized commissioning of the Breast Radiotherapy Injury Rehabilitation Service.[4]

Group 2: Moderate or mild long-term symptoms that can be self-managed and/or treated by local services/primary care

- These consequences affect a greater proportion of people (5–25% of those treated, depending on treatment type and other factors).
- They are unlikely to be identified without patient-reported outcome measures (PROMs), as they may not be reported as a 'severe toxicity', but they do have a negative impact on QOL.

Example: Bowel urgency as a consequence of pelvic cancer treatment
Bowel urgency is a common but debilitating symptom following pelvic radiotherapy, colorectal surgery and immunotherapy. Symptoms can be identified by a few validated questions,[5] and cause(s) and treatment(s) can be identified by health professionals, including GPs and nurses, through use of an evidence-based clinical algorithm.[6]

Group 3: No ongoing symptoms but an increased risk of a second primary cancer or other life-limiting condition, e.g. cardiovascular disease or osteoporosis

These 'late effects' may have little or no immediate symptomatic impact after cancer treatment, but they carry the risk of major later impact on patients' well-being and survival.

- They are relevant to the largest proportion of people.
- They may not become apparent until years after cancer treatment has ended.

Example: Chemotherapy and cardiovascular disease
Many cancer treatments, such as anthracyclines, trastuzumab and hormonal treatments, carry an increased risk of cardiovascular disease, particularly in an ageing population of cancer survivors with comorbidities and in adult survivors of childhood cancer treatment who may present with cardiovascular symptoms at a relatively young age.[7]

The GP is particularly important for this group in preventing, identifying and managing these long-term conditions.

The recovery package

The NCSI recommended each patient should have access to a recovery package:[1,8] a suite of simple interventions that can enable tailored and coordinated support for people with cancer. In England, the government and NHS England committed to everyone having access by 2020 as part of the 2015 cancer strategy[9] and the *Five year forward view*.[10] It should include a holistic needs assessment (HNA), which is an opportunity for those with cancer to discuss their physical, emotional, practical and financial needs with a health professional at critical points in their cancer journey. As a minimum, this should occur shortly after diagnosis and at the end of treatment. HNA discussions help secondary care to provide person-centred information and support to people with cancer during their treatment and beyond. The electronic HNA was developed by Macmillan Cancer Support to provide a framework for this conversation and enables issues to be raised and recorded electronically. It can then be interrogated to understand why QOL scores may be low in a particular cancer population. The treatment summary from secondary to primary care is another critical element of the recovery package. It helps to ensure that the GP and patient are aware of how treatment may affect future illness risk and therefore what action they may need to take. Another element of the package is the cancer care review in primary care. Like the HNA, it aims to provide an opportunity to understand the current needs of the patient and share information with them about what they can do to help lower their future risk, e.g. through physical activity, adopting a better diet or stopping smoking. To support primary care to provide optimal cancer care reviews, and to better support patients in the long term, Macmillan Cancer Support worked with the Royal College of General Practitioners to develop an educational resource.[11]

Addressing the consequences of treatment

The NCSI set out a three part strategy to address the issue of consequences of treatment.

- Prevent, where possible, by selecting the best possible treatment for the patient and avoiding overtreatment.
- Describe, record and report consequences that could not be prevented.
- Provide evidence-based services, guidance and information where required.

On the last point, the NCSI, and subsequently Macmillan Cancer Support, worked on two key areas.

- Service model testing focused on developing a model to manage key long-term consequences of cancer treatment symptoms. A good example of such a model is managing bowel and other symptoms after pelvic cancers. Testing and development of evidence-based gastroenterologist-led and nurse-led clinics led to expert consensus on an overall tiered service model (Figure 10.1), which covers the management of mild to severe pelvic problems in a hub-and-spoke arrangement.
- A range of guidance and resources for specialist and generalist health professionals and for people affected by cancer was produced using a three-part framework of guidance for specialists, non-specialists and people affected by cancer (Table 10.1).

Describing and reporting consequences of treatment and the QOL metric

The 2015 cancer strategy for England included a recommendation to develop a new QOL metric for cancer by 2020.[9] The role of a QOL metric is to show at a national level where cancer patients are reporting poorer QOL after treatment. To clarify the cause of poor QOL or what could be done to improve it requires additional data. Understanding the relationship between a treatment and a negative outcome requires routine collection of PROMs and more detailed QOL survey data that can describe outcomes related to particular treatments, e.g. bowel urgency.

Example: Colorectal cancer and bowel urgency

Research using patient-reported QOL measures revealed the following:

- Patients' QOL can remain poor after treatment.[38]
- If a small number of issues can explain most instances of patient-reported poor QOL, only these issues need to be asked about initially.
- Bowel urgency was shown to have a significant impact on QOL and be associated with different types and quality of treatment.
- If bowel urgency persisted or recurred a year after treatment then it was likely to be an ongoing issue for at least the next 6 years.[39]
- Identifying that someone was experiencing bowel urgency using four validated questions enabled appropriate evidence-based support/treatment to be provided to improve QOL.[5]

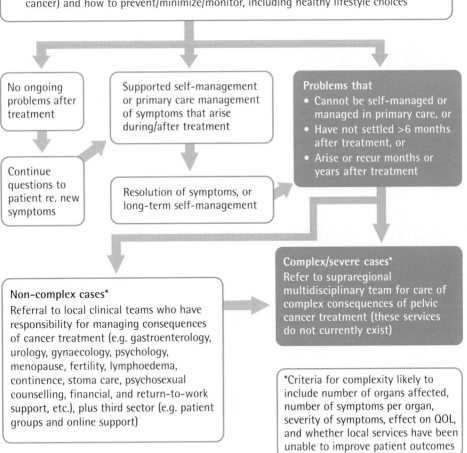

Before, during and after pelvic cancer radiotherapy/other treatments
- Provision of information and helpful resources (such as toilet card/RADAR key) to patients and carers, including tailored discussion of long-term and late-onset consequences of treatment, plus who to contact and what to do should they arise
- Systematic identification of consequences of treatment (through repeated use of HNA, PROMs or other structured questions)

At end of treatment
- HNA and care planning
- Treatment summary sent to the patient and other healthcare teams, alerting them to potential future consequences (such as cardiac problems, osteoporosis or second primary cancer) and how to prevent/minimize/monitor, including healthy lifestyle choices

No ongoing problems after treatment

Supported self-management or primary care management of symptoms that arise during/after treatment

Problems that
- Cannot be self-managed or managed in primary care, or
- Have not settled >6 months after treatment, or
- Arise or recur months or years after treatment

Continue questions to patient re. new symptoms

Resolution of symptoms, or long-term self-management

Complex/severe cases*
Refer to supraregional multidisciplinary team for care of complex consequences of pelvic cancer treatment (these services do not currently exist)

Non-complex cases*
Referral to local clinical teams who have responsibility for managing consequences of cancer treatment (e.g. gastroenterology, urology, gynaecology, psychology, menopause, fertility, lymphoedema, continence, stoma care, psychosexual counselling, financial, and return-to-work support, etc.), plus third sector (e.g. patient groups and online support)

*Criteria for complexity likely to include number of organs affected, number of symptoms per organ, severity of symptoms, effect on QOL, and whether local services have been unable to improve patient outcomes

Supported by The Royal College of Radiologists, British Society of Gastroenterology, Society of Radiographers, UK Oncology Nursing Society, Macmillan Cancer Support, Pelvic Radiation Disease Association, Bowel Cancer UK, Prostate Cancer UK, and Jo's Cervical Cancer Trust.

Figure 10.1 Tiered model for management of consequences of pelvic cancer treatments.

Table 10.1 Summary of guidance on managing the consequences of treatment for professionals and people affected by cancer.

Area of consequences of treatment	For specialists	For non-specialists	For people affected by cancer[a]
Bowel	Guidance: the practical management of gastrointestinal symptoms of pelvic radiation disease[12]	Managing lower gastrointestinal problems after cancer treatment[13]	Managing the late effects of pelvic radiotherapy in women[14] Managing the late effects of pelvic radiotherapy in men[15] Managing the late effects of bowel cancer treatment[16]
Urinary (male)	Faithfull et al.[17]		
Sexual (male)	Kirby et al.[18]	Treating erectile dysfunction after surgery for pelvic cancers[20]	Managing the late effects of pelvic radiotherapy in men[15]
	White et al.[19]	Treating erectile dysfunction after radical radiotherapy and androgen deprivation therapy (ADT) for prostate cancer[21]	Cancer and your sex life – information for men[22] Cancer treatment and fertility – information for men[23]
Upper gastrointestinal	Guidance: managing persistent upper gastrointestinal symptoms during and after treatment for cancer[24]		
Heart health		Managing heart health during and after cancer treatment[25] Tips for managing heart health during and after cancer treatment[26]	Heart health and cancer treatment[27]
Endocrine	In development by the Society for Endocrinology		
Gynaecological		Guidance on long-term consequences of treatment for gynaecological cancer (part 1: pelvic radiotherapy)[28]	Managing the late effects of pelvic radiotherapy in women[14] Cancer and your sex life – information for women[29] Cancer treatment and fertility – information for women[30]
Colorectal and anal cancer		Managing the long-term consequences of colorectal and anal cancer[31]	Managing the late effects of bowel cancer treatment[16]
Head and neck			Managing the late effects of head and neck cancer[32]
Breast			Managing the late effects of breast cancer treatment[33]
Any	A competence framework for nurses caring for people living with and beyond cancer[34] After cancer treatment: a guide for professionals[35]		What to do after cancer treatment ends: 10 top tips[36] Life after cancer treatment[37]

[a]Not exhaustive.

Summary

People living after cancer can have poor health as a consequence of their cancer or its treatment. This may require long-term monitoring, self-management or specialist services. In line with commitments made by government and NHS England, by 2020 everyone in England who has had a cancer diagnosis should have access to a recovery package, and a new QOL metric should have been embedded in the NHS. As a result, identification and awareness of the consequences of cancer and its treatment should be increased, both at the level of individual direct care through HNAs and at a national level through the metric. The provision of guidance for patients and professionals and the further development of dedicated services for people with long-term consequences of cancer treatments are therefore of great importance due to the increasing numbers of people who will be identified as having unmet needs.

References

1 Department of Health, Macmillan Cancer Support, NHS Improvement. *The National Cancer Survivorship Initiative vision.* London: Department of Health, 2010.

2 Macmillan Cancer Support (2013). *Throwing light on the consequences of cancer and its treatment.* Available from:
www.macmillan.org.uk/documents/aboutus/research/researchandevaluationreports/
throwinglightontheconsequencesofcanceranditstreatment.pdf (accessed 13 July 2017).

3 Macmillan Cancer Support (2010). *Getting it right.* Available from:
https://be.macmillan.org.uk/Downloads/ResourcesForSupporters/CampaignReports/MAC12
965-RAGE-Final-Report.pdf (accessed 9 May 2017).

4 Royal United Hospitals Bath NHS Foundation Trust. *Breast Radiotherapy Injury Rehabilitation Service.* Available from: www.rnhrd.nhs.uk/175 (accessed 9 May 2017).

5 Taylor S, Byrne A, Adams R, *et al.* The three-item ALERT-B questionnaire provides a validated screening tool to detect chronic gastrointestinal symptoms after pelvic radiotherapy in cancer survivors. *Clin Oncol (R Coll Radiol)* 2016; 28: e139–47.

6 Andreyev HJ, Muls AC, Norton C, *et al.* Guidance: the practical management of the gastrointestinal symptoms of pelvic radiation disease. *Frontline Gastroenterol* 2015; 6: 53–72.

7 Ewer MS, Ewer SM. Cardiotoxicity of anticancer treatments. *Nat Rev Cardiol* 2015; 12: 547–58.

8 Macmillan Cancer Support (2014). *The recovery package.* Available from:
www.macmillan.org.uk/about-us/health-professionals/programmes-and-services/recovery-package (accessed 9 May 2017).

9 The Independent Cancer Taskforce (2015). *Achieving world-class cancer outcomes: a strategy for England 2015–2020.* Available from:
www.cancerresearchuk.org/sites/default/files/achieving_world-class_cancer_outcomes_-
_a_strategy_for_england_2015-2020.pdf (accessed 13 July 2017).

10 NHS England (2014). *Five year forward view.* Available from: www.england.nhs.uk/wp-content/uploads/2014/10/5yfv-web.pdf (accessed 13 July 2017).

11 Royal College of General Practitioners. *Consequences of cancer and treatment.* Available from:
www.rcgp.org.uk/clinical-and-research/toolkits/consequences-of-cancer-toolkit.aspx
(accessed 13 July 2017).

12 Macmillan Cancer Support (2014). *Guidance: the practical management of gastrointestinal symptoms of pelvic radiation disease*. Available from: https://be.macmillan.org.uk/be/p-21663-guidance-the-practical-management-of-gastrointestinal-symptoms-of-pelvic-radiation-disease.aspx (accessed 13 July 2017).

13 Macmillan Cancer Support (2015). *Managing lower gastrointestinal problems after cancer treatment. A quick guide for health professionals*. Available from: https://be.macmillan.org.uk/be/p-22586-managing-lower-gastrointestinal-problems-after-cancer-treatment.aspx (accessed 13 July 2017).

14 Macmillan Cancer Support (2015). *Managing the late effects of pelvic radiotherapy in women*. Available from: https://be.macmillan.org.uk/be/p-20086-managing-the-late-effects-of-pelvic-radiotherapy-in-women.aspx (accessed 13 July 2017).

15 Macmillan Cancer Support (2015). *Managing the late effects of pelvic radiotherapy in men*. Available from: https://be.macmillan.org.uk/be/p-20085-managing-the-late-effects-of-pelvic-radiotherapy-in-men.aspx (accessed 13 July 2017).

16 Macmillan Cancer Support (2015). *Managing the late effects of bowel cancer treatment*. Available from: https://be.macmillan.org.uk/be/p-19095-managing-the-late-effects-of-bowel-cancer-treatment.aspx (accessed 13 July 2017).

17 Faithfull S, Lemanska A, Aslet P, *et al*. Integrative review on the non-invasive management of lower urinary tract symptoms in men following treatments for pelvic malignancies. *Int J Clin Pract* 2015; 69: 1184–208.

18 Kirby MG, White ID, Butcher J, *et al*. Development of UK recommendations on treatment for post-surgical erectile dysfunction. *Int J Clin Pract* 2014; 68: 590–608.

19 White ID, Wilson J, Aslet P, *et al*. Development of UK guidance on the management of erectile dysfunction resulting from radical radiotherapy and androgen deprivation therapy for prostate cancer. *Int J Clin Pract* 2015; 69: 106–23.

20 Macmillan Cancer Support (2014). *Treating erectile dysfunction after surgery for pelvic cancers*. Available from: https://be.macmillan.org.uk/be/p-22277-treating-erectile-dysfunction-after-surgery-for-pelvic-cancers.aspx (accessed 13 July 2017).

21 Macmillan Cancer Support (2014). *Treating erectile dysfunction after radical radiotherapy and androgen deprivation therapy (ADT) for prostate cancer*. Available from: https://be.macmillan.org.uk/be/p-22276-treating-erectile-dysfunction-after-radical-radiotherapy.aspx (accessed 13 July 2017).

22 Macmillan Cancer Support (2016). *Cancer and your sex life – information for men*. Available from: https://be.macmillan.org.uk/be/p-21634-cancer-and-your-sex-life-information-for-men.aspx (accessed 13 July 2017).

23 Macmillan Cancer Support (2016). *Cancer treatment and fertility – information for men*. Available from: https://be.macmillan.org.uk/be/p-690-cancer-treatment-and-fertility-information-for-men.aspx (accessed 13 July 2017).

24 Macmillan Cancer Support (2015). *Guidance: managing persistent upper gastrointestinal symptoms during and after treatment for cancer*. Available from: https://be.macmillan.org.uk/be/p-23613-guidance-managing-persistent-upper-gastrointestinal-symptoms.aspx (accessed 13 July 2017).

25 Macmillan Cancer Support (2015). *Managing heart health during and after cancer treatment. A quick guide for primary care health professionals.*. Available from: https://be.macmillan.org.uk/be/p-22855-managing-heart-health-during-and-after-cancer-treatment-guide.aspx (accessed 13 July 2017).

26 Macmillan Cancer Support (2014). *Tips for managing heart health during and after cancer treatment.* Available from: www.macmillan.org.uk/_images/managing-heart-health-quick-tips-guide_tcm9-297838.pdf (accessed 13 July 2017).

27 Macmillan Cancer Support (2017). *Heart health and cancer treatment.* Available from: https://be.macmillan.org.uk/be/p-22060-heart-health-and-cancer-treatment.aspx (accessed 13 July 2017).

28 Macmillan Cancer Support (2014). *Guidance on long-term consequences of treatment for gynaecological cancer (part 1: pelvic radiotherapy).* Available from: https://be.macmillan.org.uk/be/p-21594-guidance-on-long-term-consequences-of-treatment-for-gynaecological-cancer.aspx (accessed 13 July 2017).

29 Macmillan Cancer Support (2016). *Cancer and your sex life – information for women.* Available from: https://be.macmillan.org.uk/be/p-21635-cancer-and-your-sex-life-information-for-women.aspx (accessed 13 July 2017).

30 Macmillan Cancer Support (2016). *Cancer treatment and fertility – information for women.* Available from: https://be.macmillan.org.uk/be/p-691-cancer-treatment-and-fertility-information-for-women.aspx (accessed 13 July 2017).

31 Macmillan Cancer Support (2015). *Managing the long term consequences of colorectal and anal cancer.* Available from: https://be.macmillan.org.uk/be/p-23019-managing-the-long-term-consequences-of-colorectal-and-anal-cancer.aspx (accessed 13 July 2017).

32 Macmillan Cancer Support (2016). *Managing the late effects of head and neck cancer.* Available from: https://be.macmillan.org.uk/be/p-21571-managing-the-late-effects-of-head-and-neck-cancer.aspx (accessed 13 July 2017).

33 Macmillan Cancer Support (2016). *Managing the late effects of breast cancer treatment.* Available from: https://be.macmillan.org.uk/be/p-19078-managing-the-late-effects-of-breast-cancer-treatment.aspx (accessed 13 July 2017).

34 Macmillan Cancer Support (2014). *A competence framework for nurses caring for people living with and beyond cancer.* Available from: https://be.macmillan.org.uk/be/p-21583-a-competence-framework-for-nurses.aspx (accessed 13 July 2017).

35 Macmillan Cancer Support (2014). *After cancer treatment: a guide for professionals.* Available from: https://be.macmillan.org.uk/be/p-21036-after-cancer-treatment-a-guide-for-professionals.aspx (accessed 13 July 2017).

36 Macmillan Cancer Support (2017). *What to do after cancer treatment ends: 10 top tips.* Available from: https://be.macmillan.org.uk/be/p-20338-what-to-do-after-cancer-treatment-ends-10-top-tips.aspx (accessed 13 July 2017).

37 Macmillan Cancer Support (2014). *Life after cancer treatment.* Available from: https://be.macmillan.org.uk/be/p-18826-life-after-cancer-treatment.aspx (accessed 13 July 2017).

38 Glaser AW, Fraser LK, Corner J, *et al.* Patient-reported outcomes of cancer survivors in England 1–5 years after diagnosis: a cross-sectional survey. *BMJ Open* 2013; 3: e002317.

39 Adams E, Boulton MG, Horne A, *et al.* The effects of pelvic radiotherapy on cancer survivors: symptom profile, psychological morbidity and quality of life. *Clin Oncol* 2014; 26: 10–17.

11 Integration of Palliative Care Support into Oncology Practice

Lucy Ziegler, Michael I. Bennett

Introduction

Scientific advances have led to ever-increasing cancer treatment options and longer lives for patients with incurable malignancies. Many of these patients have complex symptoms due to the cumulative effects of long-term cancer treatment, disease progression and pre-existing morbidities. There is a need for efficacious supportive care interventions aimed at relieving the debilitating physical and psychological symptoms which have a negative impact on quality of life (QOL).[1] The advances in cancer treatment have outpaced progress in terms of supportive care provision for cancer patients, and only in the last decade has palliative care become recognized as an essential component of oncology care and integrated models of care have been proposed and evaluated. The World Health Organization defines palliative care as an approach that improves the QOL of patients and their families facing the problems associated with life-threatening illness, through the prevention and relief of suffering by means of early identification and impeccable assessment and treatment of pain and other problems, physical, psychosocial and spiritual.[2] There is a growing body of evidence to demonstrate the value of integrating palliative care into routine oncology care.[1,3–8] This chapter presents an overview of the research evidence, the patient and service level barriers to implementation, and recommendations for practice.

Recent developments

Traditionally patients with cancer were referred to palliative care as a last resort when treatment options had been exhausted and death was imminent. Over the last decade there has been a growing body of research to support earlier integration of palliative care into oncology care. The research evidence consists of a number of randomized controlled trials, largely from North America, which have demonstrated an association of early palliative care with improved symptoms and QOL and reduced acute hospital admissions and aggressive cancer treatments at the end of life.[1,3,5,7,8] The interventions in these trials varied and some of the benefits have been inconsistent across trials (e.g. QOL, symptom improvement). In general, however, common characteristics were assessment and several follow-up consultations by specialist palliative care teams over a period of 2–3 months, which occurred about 6–14 months before patients died. Systematic reviews and pooled analyses of routinely collected data have also demonstrated an association between early palliative care intervention and an increased proportion of home deaths as well as a reduction in emergency admissions for patient with cancer.[9,10] This evidence has begun to influence policy in the USA: the American Society of Clinical Oncology recommends that the integration of palliative care into oncology management should be considered early in the course of illness for any patient with metastatic cancer or a high symptom burden.[11]

Implementing this evidence in routine clinical practice in the UK presents challenges. Only two-thirds of cancer patients are referred to palliative care services before they die, and those who do receive palliative care are typically referred late in the course of their illness (median 37 days before death).[12] This is a much shorter duration of palliative care involvement than US research evidence suggests is optimal. Developing models of palliative care integration that maximize patient benefit and fit within existing service constraints is a current priority.

Oncologists play a vital role in the process of integration of palliative care. Timely integration is reliant on the oncologist's ability to determine the appropriate time to refer a patient and communicate the potential benefits of palliative care effectively, i.e. addressing any misconceptions or lack of awareness the patient or the family may have about the role of palliative care.[13] Determining the right time to refer is difficult. Although the research evidence reports patient benefits in relation to referral at specific time points before death or at diagnosis with advanced disease, this information is not easy to put into operation in clinical practice. Referring all patients at diagnosis with advanced disease is not currently feasible in routine practice: the palliative care services would be overburdened and not all patients at diagnosis with advanced disease have complex symptoms or are receptive to a palliative care referral. Determining an accurate time from death even in patients with cancers that have a relatively predictable prognosis is challenging. Studies have shown that medical oncologists' estimates of life expectancy in newly referred patients with incurable cancer are imprecise: 29% were within 0.67–1.33 times the actual survival time, 35% were too optimistic (>1.33 times the actual survival time) and 39% were too pessimistic (<0.67 times the actual survival time).[14] It may be that the reason some patients are referred to palliative care close to death or not at all is in part related to these prognostic challenges.

Barriers to timely referral to palliative care also exist at a health professional level. Studies exploring cancer professionals' views about integration of palliative care have found that although they acknowledge the importance of timely referral they recognize that, in reality, referral often does not occur until a patient is very obviously nearing the end of life or experiences an acute episode.[15] The explanations oncologists offered for why referrals are not made before this point include attempting to delay the termination of active treatment, feeling that they were abandoning the patient, difficulty initiating the conversation about palliative care, and feeling ill equipped to deal with end-of-life issues.[16] Emphasis on more training in palliative care in the oncology training curriculum and increasing continued medical education on this topic are important.

Society's views on palliative care are another factor that influences prompt integration of palliative care into oncology care. Studies exploring patient barriers to referral to palliative care report misconceptions regarding the role of hospices and Macmillan nurses, which included assumptions that palliative care was only for patients at the very end of life, and a lack of appreciation of the breadth of services provided.[10] The prevalent misconceptions reported in these studies suggest that the nature of palliative care services should be explained in more detail when first introduced and that information materials should be provided to reinforce understanding.

Conclusion

Evidence clearly supports the benefits to patients of earlier referral to palliative care, but the challenge for clinical services and researchers is how to put this into operation in routine care. A starting point is to promote more widely the concept of earlier integration of palliative care into oncology management, rather than handing over once all oncology options have been exhausted. Defining and promoting palliative care interventions so that they are perceived as enhancing patients' lives would be an important step forward and help to counter the perception that referral represents oncological failure or imminent death; for example, highlighting expertise in symptom control, psychological support for patients and families, and support for discussions about the nature and place of future care should the cancer progress. Developing patient support materials and more integrated clinical practices such as joint oncology and palliative care clinics would help to underpin these concepts.

References

1 Greer JA, Jackson VA, Meier DE, Temel JS. Early integration of palliative care services with standard oncology care for patients with advanced cancer. *CA Cancer J Clin* 2013; 63: 349–63.

2 World Health Organization. *National cancer control programmes: policies and managerial guidelines.* 2nd ed. Geneva: WHO, 2002.

3 Zimmermann C, Swami N, Krzyzanowska M, *et al.* Early palliative care for patients with advanced cancer: a cluster-randomised controlled trial. *Lancet* 2014; 383: 1721–30.

4 Glare PA. Early implementation of palliative care can improve patient outcomes. *J Natl Compr Canc Netw* 2013; 11 (suppl 1): S3–9.

5 Bakitas MA, Tosteson TD, Li Z, *et al.* Early versus delayed initiation of concurrent palliative oncology care: patient outcomes in the ENABLE III randomized controlled trial. *J Clin Oncol* 2015; 33: 1438–45.

6 Bauman JR, Temel JS. The integration of early palliative care with oncology care: the time has come for a new tradition. *J Natl Compr Canc Netw* 2014; 12: 1763–71.

7 Rugno FC, Paiva BS, Paiva CE. Early integration of palliative care facilitates the discontinuation of anticancer treatment in women with advanced breast or gynecologic cancers. *Gynecol Oncol* 2014; 135: 249–54.

8 Temel JS, Greer JA, Muzikansky A, *et al.* Early palliative care for patients with metastatic non-small-cell lung cancer. *N Engl J Med* 2010; 363: 733–42.

9 Henson L, Gao W, Higginson I, *et al.* Emergency department attendance by patients with cancer in the last month of life: a systematic review and meta-analysis. *Lancet* 2015; 385 (suppl 1): S41.

10 Seow H, Brazil K, Sussman J, *et al.* Impact of community based, specialist palliative care teams on hospitalisations and emergency department visits late in life and hospital deaths: a pooled analysis. *BMJ* 2014; 348: g3496.

11 Smith TJ, Temin S, Alesi ER, *et al.* American Society of Clinical Oncology provisional clinical opinion: the integration of palliative care into standard oncology care. *J Clin Oncol* 2012; 30: 880–7.

12 Bennett MI, Ziegler L, Allsop M, *et al.* What determines duration of palliative care before death for patients with advanced disease? A retrospective cohort study of community and hospital palliative care provision in a large UK city. *BMJ Open* 2016; 6: e012576.

13 Johnson LA, Gorman C, Morse R, *et al.* Does communication skills training make a difference to patients' experiences of consultations in oncology and palliative care services? *Eur J Cancer Care (Engl)* 2013; 22: 202–9.

14 Stockler MR, Tattersall MH, Boyer MJ, *et al.* Disarming the guarded prognosis: predicting survival in newly referred patients with incurable cancer. *Br J Cancer* 2006; 94: 208–12.

15 Johnson C, Girgis A, Paul C, *et al.* Australian palliative care providers' perceptions and experiences of the barriers and facilitators to palliative care provision. *Support Care Cancer* 2011; 19: 343–51.

16 Charalambous H, Pallis A, Hasan B, O'Brien M. Attitudes and referral patterns of lung cancer specialists in Europe to specialized palliative care (SPC) and the practice of early palliative care (EPC). *BMC Palliat Care* 2014; 13: 59.

12 Integration of Supportive Care into Oncology Clinics Ensures Best Practice for Patients with Metastatic Cancer

Tracey Coleby, Lorraine Turner, Andrew M. Wardley

Introduction

The multidisciplinary team (MDT) meeting has been the cornerstone of cancer care over the last two decades and has been shown to improve survival for cancer patients.[1] The majority of MDT meetings are centred on initial diagnosis and surgical care. Over a similar time period there have been many advances in systemic anticancer therapy (SACT) for patients with advanced cancer, which have improved overall survival and quality of life (QOL). The large number of new treatments significantly increases the complexity and challenge for oncologists.[2] There is currently debate about the utility of the MDT meeting and the use of SACT in patients with metastatic disease.[3] We describe work, developed in metastatic breast cancer but applicable to other cancers, that attempts to address these two issues.

Metastatic breast cancer, being a heterogeneous biological process, exhibits a varied and unpredictable response to treatment.[2] Patients can have varying amounts and aggressiveness of disease, from minimal to extensive and slow-growing disease to rapidly progressive disease. The beneficial and harmful effects of treatment must be carefully balanced and regularly reviewed. Often during the active treatment phase, discussions around prognosis, goals of care, advance care planning and wishes for the future are seen as inappropriate and are not addressed until the patient is clearly at the end of life.

Recent developments

In an audit carried out at The Christie NHS Foundation Trust in the early 2000s we found that few patients being actively treated for metastatic breast cancer, with numerous lines of palliative SACT, had been identified as being in the last year of life. Furthermore, they had often become separated from support in the community. Consequently, admissions for supportive and terminal care were frequent. The experience of patients not accessing supportive care until they are nearing the end of life, possibly due to the negative connotations associated with palliative care, has previously been reported.[2] Patients with a high symptom burden were poorly catered for in oncology clinics, occupying considerable time and many staff.[2] Fifty-seven percent of breast care nurses report that they are unable to provide adequate provision of care for patients with metastatic breast cancer.[4] Their expertise is around helping support patients undergoing treatment, from surgery through to chemotherapy, providing physical and psychological support and signposting to other services as needed; many feel inadequate to manage patients with progressive disease.[4] It is vital that, alongside breast care nursing support, these patients receive specialist support from palliative/supportive care professionals who are skilled in managing patients with advancing disease.[5] At The Christie we developed an advanced breast cancer MDT which includes an advanced nurse practitioner in supportive care as well as breast care and research nurses, and medical oncologists. This has greatly improved patient and staff experience and has improved health resource use and trial recruitment. The fulcrum is a metastatic breast cancer MDT meeting, where all new and current patients with progressive disease on treatment are discussed and potential treatment plans, including research options, formulated. This also serves as an educational environment for medical oncology specialist training. Integration of specialist supportive care from diagnosis onwards greatly improves the management of disease and the symptoms and side effects of treatment, and promotes the best QOL possible. In addition to improving QOL, early integration of supportive care has been shown to increase survival in some patients and promote less aggressive disease management towards the end of life.[5] Furthermore, supportive care as an integral part of oncology management helps support clinicians and patients in transition from active treatment to best supportive care.[6]

The integration of supportive care into oncology evolved into enhanced supportive care, developed at The Christie to include three other disease teams, and subsequently into successful NHS England commissioning for quality and innovation (CQUIN) across 23 cancer centres.[7] The demonstrable benefits of enhanced supportive care include the following:

· Less need for hospital admissions, especially emergency admissions.
· Reduction in length of stay.
· Fewer intensive care hospital days.
· Lower overall healthcare costs, including expenditure on high-cost SACT.
· Reduced mortality within 30 days on SACT.
· Increased trial recruitment.

We have also demonstrated a reduction in patients with performance status (PS) ≥ 2 receiving SACT. A second NHS England CQUIN focuses on decisions to start and continue SACT for patients with poor PS or those commencing second line and subsequent treatments with non-curative intent.[8] The aim of the CQUIN is to better support clinicians and patients to make treatment decisions.

Within breast oncology at The Christie we have extended collaborative work and introduced an advanced nurse practitioner in experimental medicine to the whole disease group, promoting the same multidisciplinary approach for patients with metastatic breast cancer. As conventional SACT fails to benefit many patients, the opportunity to access novel therapies gives hope as well as potentially effective treatments to patients with a good PS. Earlier identification of patients for whom standard therapy is failing, providing specialist supportive care input, holistic needs assessment (HNA) and advance care planning, and identifying experimental medicine trial opportunities, has greatly increased access for patients in breast clinical oncology (from zero to four referrals per month) to new, potentially effective treatments.

As a patient's disease advances, it becomes increasingly important for healthcare professionals to be open and honest with them and their family regarding the prognosis, allowing them to make informed decisions around their wishes and prevent them undergoing futile treatments.[9] Denying patients this can prevent them from preparing for their own mortality, reflection and saying goodbye to their loved ones.[10] In their last year of life, patients have a higher level of need and require care from skilled healthcare professionals.[6]

At The Christie we have been working closely with the Manchester Macmillan Cancer Improvement Partnership in developing best practice for patients with advancing metastatic breast cancer. To date, the recommendations are that all patients should have access to a breast care nurse and be offered an HNA. Those who are symptomatic or who have advancing disease and are likely to be in their last year of life should also receive specialist supportive care alongside their breast care nursing support. Patients with progression after second line treatment should be discussed at either the MDT meeting or with another colleague to ensure appropriate, ongoing management and support. All patients should also be considered for trials, if appropriate. GPs and community teams should be informed about patients who are likely to be in their last year of life. Ensuring patients are added to the Gold Standards Framework or palliative register within the community and monitored prevents crisis intervention as they deteriorate.

Conclusion

Patients with metastatic breast cancer have complex disease and high levels of need which require a multidisciplinary approach to ensure that appropriate care and support are provided throughout the disease journey. Integrating palliative/supportive care alongside breast oncology has promoted a proactive, holistic approach to patient care, with better identification of advancing disease, ensuring increased support in the last year of life. Patients in whom subsequent conventional SACT is unlikely to be beneficial are offered the opportunity to take part in appropriate clinical trials. Improved care and support in the hospital and community settings should help to improve patient satisfaction and QOL, and prevent the need for crisis intervention.

References

1 Kesson EM, Allardice GM, George WD, *et al*. Effects of multidisciplinary team working on breast cancer survival: retrospective, comparative, interventional cohort study of 13,722 women. *BMJ* 2012; 344: e2718.

2 Reed E, Corner J. Defining the illness trajectory of metastatic breast cancer. *BMJ Support Palliat Care* 2015; 5: 358–65.

3 Tacca O, LeHeurteur M, Durando X, *et al*. Metastatic breast cancer: overall survival related to successive chemotherapies. What do we gain after the third line? *Cancer Invest* 2009; 27: 81–5.

4 Reed E, Scanlon K, Fenlon D. A survey of provision of breast care nursing for patients with metastatic breast cancer – implications for the role. *Eur J Cancer Care* 2010; 19: 575–80.

5 Temel JS, Greer JA, Muzikansky A, *et al*. Early palliative care for patients with metastatic non-small-cell lung cancer. *N Engl J Med* 2010; 363: 733–42.

6 Farrell C, Coleby T. An integrated model for breast cancer and palliative care. *Cancer Nurs Pract* 2016; 15: 28–31.

7 NHS England (2016). *Enhanced supportive care: integrating supportive care in oncology. Phase I: treatment with palliative intent*. Available from: www.england.nhs.uk/wp-content/uploads/2016/03/ca1-enhncd-supprtv-care-guid.pdf (accessed 20 March 2017).

8 NHS England (2017). CA-3 – Optimising palliative chemotherapy decision making. Available from: www.england.nhs.uk/wp-content/uploads/2016/11/ca3-optimis-palliative-chemo-decisions.pdf (accessed 20 March 2017).

9 Fallowfield LJ, Hall A, Maguire GP, Baum M. Psychological outcomes of difference treatment policies of women with early breast cancer outside a clinical trial. *BMJ* 1990; 301: 575–80.

10 Bakhurst D. On lying and deceiving. *J Med Ethics* 1992; 18: 63–6.

13 Integration of Cancer Care between Primary Care and Hospitals

Peter Selby, Geoff Hall, Ladislav Dusek, Fotios Loupakis, Lucio Luzzatto, Tit Albreht, Richard D. Neal, Rob Turner, Sean Duffy

Introduction

Despite encouraging progress, outcomes for cancer patients are still patchy and inequalities are apparent even across Europe.[1-3] Integrated cancer care, bringing together primary care and hospital care and forming closer links between institutions, can improve the quality of care and outcomes for patients.[4] This chapter summarizes approaches to improving integration between primary care and hospital services and between hospitals and other cancer services through cancer networks.

Integrating primary care with oncology and other hospital care teams

A high standard of primary care is key to the entire path of a cancer patient: from early diagnosis to the support of survivors or to terminal care. Increasingly, treatments can be delivered without hospital admissions.[4] Early diagnosis improves clinical outcomes and may reduce overall service costs.[5-8] Low public awareness of symptoms that may indicate cancer, and negative beliefs about cancer outcomes, contribute to delayed presentation, advanced stage and lower survival. Nationally coordinated, multi-component public awareness campaigns can positively influence cancer outcomes.[9]

Danish investigators have studied generic and disease-specific issues underlying delay in diagnosis. They have characterized the potential for adverse consequences from gatekeeper practices in primary care, the prevalence of cancer alarm symptoms, the impact on patients' confidence in their GP, and comparisons in the international benchmarking programmes. Their work has underpinned consensus statements such as the Aarhus statement on improving design and reporting studies on early cancer diagnosis.[10] In 2007, having recognized the lack of progress in the previous decade, the Danish government launched a new diagnostic strategy, the key components of which were that a diagnostic suspicion of cancer should be dealt with as an acute condition, with only medically necessary delays. Multidisciplinary working groups were established to describe the ideal clinical pathway for cancer types, with clear maximum acceptable waiting times and GP access to diagnostic investigations. Preliminary results are encouraging.[11]

Integrated cancer services can strengthen both vertical links between primary, secondary, tertiary and social care services for patients with cancer and horizontal links between cancer services and other hospital specialties, including diagnostic services, across all medical specialities. Comorbidities in oncology patients require that their management be shared with professionals in other specialties, e.g. cardiology, respiratory medicine, gastroenterology and especially geriatrics. On the other hand, in a cancer patient acute complications of the cancer itself or complications of its treatment may require urgent or emergency care: this highlights the need for close integration of cancer services with critical care services and with acute medical and surgical services (Figure 13.1).

Health informatics and telemedicine solutions can now be deployed within integrated healthcare models to effectively link all relevant electronic patient records and the datasets contained with them. Optimal information flow can ensure excellence in cancer care and improved patient knowledge, participation, engagement and empowerment. It also supports timely access to care and cost-effective and financially sustainable monitoring and follow-up services. Maximizing the quality and safety of follow-up care provided within the community will also minimize the duration of hospital admissions.

Key factors in the successful integration of cancer services include the following:

- Excellent multidisciplinary cancer care.
- Agreed and respected evidence-based pathways of care.
- Shared ownership of systems by patients and professionals in primary care, in hospitals and in public health; co-production of new initiatives.
- Commitment and engagement by healthcare professionals in all sectors.
- Patient engagement in service development.
- Excellent communications.
- Integrated information systems.
- Governance clearly shared.
- Routes to access service commissioners/payers.
- Research and innovation intertwined with patient care.
- Transparency and commitment to delivering and publishing outcomes.

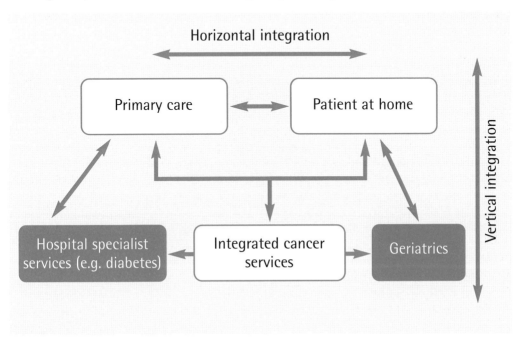

Figure 13.1 Model for integrated cancer care.

Integrating cancer care between healthcare institutions: comprehensive cancer care networks

Since the Calman–Hine report[12] and evidence reviewed in the mid-1990s,[13] structured collaboration among healthcare providers in the form of networks is increasingly recognized as a valid option for accessing and delivering high-quality specialized cancer services. This has been recently explored in considerable detail and updated by the EU Joint Action on Cancer Control (CanCon).[14] Currently, cancer care and control may be organized in different ways in different countries and regions, being influenced by history, population size and density, population distribution, health system structure and resources. In most systems there is room for improvement. In Europe many cancer patients are treated in general hospitals and/or specialized cancer institutions known as comprehensive cancer centres. A consistent and broadly applicable definition of a comprehensive cancer centre does not exist, but the Organisation of European Cancer Institutes in its voluntary accreditation procedure lays emphasis on a wide range of elements, including infrastructure for cancer care, human resources, clinical care activities, research activities, education and institutional structure.[15] Adequate patient volumes to ensure the presence of specialized multidisciplinary teams for all cancers is a feature of such centres and is associated with improved outcomes in many cases.[16–18]

Integrated cancer control and cancer care networks seek to ensure prompt access to local cancer services for diagnosis and many aspects of care, together with ready access to high-volume specialized centres for appropriate care when needed, thus aiming to achieve care quality on a par with that of a comprehensive cancer centre. Network models are attractive in principle because by fostering communication and collaboration they can both draw on the experience and abilities of the constituent units, thus implementing synergies, and significantly reduce geographical inequalities by having multiple entry points and offering cancer control services to the entire population living within an area. The EU CanCon guide outlines a highly integrated network, the comprehensive cancer care network (CCCN) (Table 13.1, Figure 13.2), and reviews how CCCNs can be planned and established, how they work and what purpose they serve.[14]

Results from a 2015 survey of EU member states indicated that cancer networks do exist in many countries, as institutions share expertise and facilities for cancer services.[14] Networks can adopt various configurations that may fit the context of individual countries. The survey suggested that the notion of integrated cancer networks (whether at national or regional level or whether with a hub and spoke pattern) is gaining ground in response to the needs of contemporary oncology. Given the apparent relationships between service volumes and outcomes,[16,17] it is suggested that a CCCN should serve a population of at least 1–2 million people.[14] Staffing is a major contributor to both processes and outcomes and is key to the success of a network. Measuring the performance and quality of cancer care services and programmes is essential to ensure that objectives are being met. It is necessary to have information technology systems to support improvements in cancer control in the network, with clear legal and administrative frameworks for the collection, sharing and reporting of data.

A CCCN is an integrated structure bridging different care sectors such as primary, secondary, tertiary and social care. Bringing links between primary care and cancer services is clearly critically important for timely access to the best treatment. However, integration between cancer services and non-cancer hospital services is equally important in modern practice, as discussed above. Cancer networks cannot, therefore, be developed separately from general healthcare services, and integration with a general healthcare service is a particular

Table 13.1 Definition of a CCCN.

- A CCCN consists of multiple units belonging to different institutions dedicated to research, prevention, diagnosis, treatment, follow-up, supportive and palliative care, and rehabilitation for the benefit of cancer patients and cancer survivors. The key elements defining a CCCN are illustrated in Figure 13.2

- These units interact and have a formal agreement to work together in a programmatic and structured way, with common governance, in order to pursue their goals more effectively and efficiently through collective synergies

- Within the CCCN the care of patients is the responsibility of inter-professional teams that are multidisciplinary and tumour-specific. Each team or tumour management group works together for the benefit of patients with that particular type of tumour

- Within the CCCN all units work together and adopt uniform standards of care for cancer-specific pathways that are binding for the entire network

- The CCCN promotes a uniform system of quality assurance, and a unified informatics system for optimal exchange of information

- The objective of a CCCN is to provide comprehensive cancer care to all people living in a certain geographic area, thus pursuing equality and the improvement of outcomes and quality

The word unit is used to designate any component of a CCCN, whether an entire pre-existing institution or part of an institution. For example, a unit might be an entire cancer centre, an oncology department of a general hospital or a children's hospital, a mammography facility, a pathology laboratory carrying out mutation analysis, or a hospice.

challenge for single-specialty cancer hospitals, which are still an important part of cancer services throughout Europe.

Creating a CCCN in Czechia (formerly the Czech Republic): a CanCon pilot project[14]

The project set out to optimize the care of every cancer patient in the target region. South Moravia and Vysočina (approximately 1.6 million people) were identified to have appropriate demographic and epidemiological characteristics. One purpose of the pilot was to verify that contractual agreements among network elements, structured collaboration with common governance, a common database encapsulating a unified patient information and quality assurance system – all characteristic of a CCCN – were compatible with full respect for established institutions. Multiple access points to the network are controlled to help patients receive timely treatment of equally high quality wherever they live. All methodologies used and progress made are fully reflected in two web portals (see below). The principles were as follows:

- A voluntary decision of healthcare providers.
- Pre-existing cancer care facilities were not removed but improved.
- A legal framework supported institutional participation and centralized data handling.
- Hospital diagnostic centres, primary care providers and palliative care units were all involved and facilitated by a common information system and research and educational facilities.
- A legally binding agreement defined its organization and governance.
- A shared system of multidisciplinary tumour management teams, common clinical protocols and a common information system and database supported unified quality assurance.

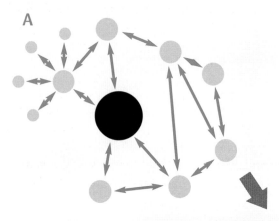

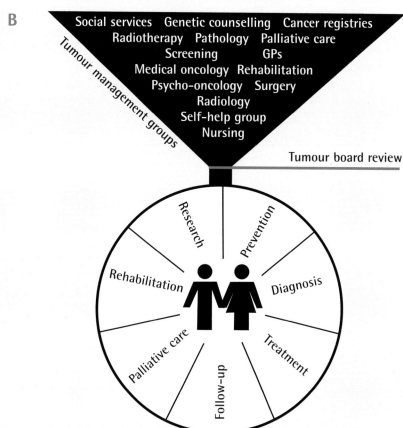

Figure 13.2 The key elements defining a CCCN. (A) Network: the dots represent units/institutions (e.g. primary care, community hospitals, university hospitals, psychosocial counselling) dedicated to research, prevention, diagnosis, treatment, follow-up, supportive and palliative care, and rehabilitation, which work together as a CCCN in a structured way with a common governance. (B) Functionality: the tumour management groups within the CCCN are inter-professional, multidisciplinary and tumour-specific, with the objective to provide comprehensive cancer care to all people living in a certain geographic area.

- The objectives of the information system included the identification of inequalities, feedback control of effectiveness, and population-based quantification of outcomes using uniform performance indicators.

The CCCN pilot is supported by two key interactive web portals.

- A national portal (www.onconet.cz) centred on cancer care management that maps infrastructures and facilitates navigation for both public and professionals.
- A web portal (cccn.onconet.cz/index.php) that outlines and details the structure of the CCCN and the rules according to which it operates, and charts patient pathways and standards for outcome measures.

The CCCN team will measure improved equity of standardized care, improved continuity of cancer care pathways and adherence to shared protocols. Initial experience suggests that the cancer network may achieve the following:

- Improve equity in access to good-quality care near home.
- Implement a patient-centred approach to common principles, attitudes and management protocols.
- Acquire resources that an individual hospital may not, and allocate them efficiently, thus avoiding duplication.
- Capitalize on complementary expertise of individual professionals for planning.
- Provide a seamless care pathway, even for patients requiring complex treatment. This may require that parts of some treatment plans are delivered at different institutions, with the CCCN ensuring that care does not become disjointed and key clinical information is always readily available.
- Be closer to primary care or fully integrated with it.
- Gather optimal conditions to conduct research.

Conclusion

There is good evidence that prompt diagnosis and specialized multidisciplinary care bring substantial benefits to cancer patients, and that integration of primary, secondary, tertiary and social care, and integration into networks of healthcare institutions, can help us to deliver care in an effective, equitable and inclusive way. New developments in health informatics give us additional tools to help us work together. Despite recognition of the value of an integrated approach through cancer networks for over two decades, there remains a great deal of work to do to deliver these benefits to all patients.

References

1   European Cancer Patient Coalition (2015). *Challenging the Europe of disparities in cancer. A framework for improved survival and better quality of life for European cancer patients.* Available from:
    www.ecpc.org/Documents/Policy&Advocacy/Europe%20of%20Disparities/Europe%20of%20 Disparities%2027th%20Sept%202015.pdf (accessed 20 July 2017).

2   Lawler M, Banks M, Law K, *et al.* The European Cancer Patient's Bill of Rights, update and implementation 2016. *ESMO Open* 2016; 1: e000127.

3   Allemani C, Weir HK and Carreira H, *et al.* Global surveillance of cancer survival 1995–2009: analysis of individual data for 25,676,887 patients from 279 population-based registries in 67 countries (CONCORD-2). *Lancet* 2015; 385: 977–1010.

4 Rubin G, Berendsen A, Crawford SM, *et al.* The expanding role of primary care in cancer control. *Lancet Oncol* 2015; 16: 1231–72.

5 Neal RD, Tharmanathan P, France B, *et al.* Is increased time to diagnosis and treatment in symptomatic cancer associated with poorer outcomes? Systematic review. *Br J Cancer* 2015; 112 (suppl 1): S92–107.

6 Cancer Research UK (2014). Saving lives, averting costs. An analysis of the financial implications of achieving earlier diagnosis of colorectal, lung and ovarian cancer. Available from: www.cancerresearchuk.org/sites/default/files/saving_lives_averting_costs.pdf (accessed 20 July 2017).

7 Rubin G, Walter F, Emery J, *et al.* Research into practice: prompt diagnosis of cancer in primary care. *Br J Gen Pract* 2014; 64: 428–30.

8 Hiom SC. Diagnosing cancer earlier: reviewing the evidence for improving cancer survival. *Br J Cancer* 2015; 112 (suppl 1): S1–5.

9 Ironmonger L, Ohuma E, Ormiston-Smith N, *et al.* An evaluation of the impact of large-scale interventions to raise public awareness of a lung cancer symptom. *Br J Cancer* 2015; 112: 207–16.

10 Weller D, Vedsted P, Rubin G, *et al.* The Aarhus statement: improving design and reporting of studies on early cancer diagnosis. *Br J Cancer* 2012; 106: 1262–7.

11 Jensen H, Tørring ML, Olesen F, *et al.* Diagnostic intervals before and after implementation of cancer patient pathways – a GP survey and registry based comparison of three cohorts of cancer patients. *BMC Cancer* 2015; 15: 308.

12 Calman K, Hine D. *A policy framework for commissioning cancer services. A report by the Expert Advisory Group on Cancer to the chief medical officers of England and Wales.* London: Department of Health, 1995.

13 Selby P, Gillis C, Haward R. Benefits from specialised cancer care. *Lancet* 1996; 348: 313–18.

14 Albreht T, Amati C, Angelastro A, *et al.* Integrated cancer control: the case for comprehensive cancer care networks (CCCN). In: Albreht T, Kiasuwa T, Van den Bulcke M, eds. *European guide on quality improvement in comprehensive cancer control.* Ljubljana: National Institute of Public Health, 2017.

15 Saghatchian M, Hummel H, Otter R, *et al.* Towards quality, comprehensiveness and excellence. The accreditation project of the Organisation of European Cancer Institutes (OECI). *Tumori* 2008; 94: 164–71.

16 Trinh QD, Bjartell A, Freedland SJ, *et al.* A systematic review of the volume–outcome relationship for radical prostatectomy. *Eur Urol* 2013; 64: 786–98.

17 Lüchtenborg M, Riaz SP, Coupland VH, *et al.* High procedure volume is strongly associated with improved survival after lung cancer surgery. *J Clin Oncol* 2013; 31: 3141–6.

18 Tremblay D, Touati N, Roberge D, *et al.* Understanding cancer networks better to implement them more effectively: a mixed methods multi-case study. *Implement Sci* 2016; 11: 39.

14 Psychosexual Difficulties after Cancer

Isabel White, Justin Grayer

Introduction

Prevalence rates of sexual difficulties associated with cancer and its treatment vary widely depending on the primary diagnosis, treatment modality, method(s) of assessment and threshold criteria for severity and type of sexual dysfunction. Rates generally exceed those found in the general UK adult population of 14.1% (in the 16–24 year age group) to 27.8% (in the 55–64 year age group).[1] This national population survey of sexual lifestyles and attitudes also found a strong association between low sexual function and age >55 years, menopause, depression, poor self-assessed general health and relationship satisfaction; these are also relevant factors for those affected by cancer.[1]

Sexual consequences following cancer treatment are common, particularly among people treated for pelvic malignancies or breast cancer, with over 50% experiencing severe and persistent disruption to their sexual well-being.[2] Given the biopsychosocial aetiology of many sexual difficulties, the increased use of nerve-sparing surgery and targeted pelvic radiotherapy techniques may not directly translate into reduced rates of sexual dysfunction. Furthermore, primary chemoradiotherapy for gynaecological or anal cancer and extended endocrine therapy (especially aromatase inhibitors) for breast cancer also contribute significantly to the high rates and severity of sexual disruption seen in oncology.[3] Common treatment-associated sexual difficulties include loss of sexual interest, arousal and sexual pain difficulties, orgasmic or ejaculatory difficulties, and reduced sexual confidence and satisfaction.

In women, sexual consequences may arise from premature menopause with reduced vaginal lubrication and dyspareunia (sexual pain), orgasmic difficulties and reduced sexual satisfaction. Pelvic surgery, radiotherapy and vaginal graft versus host disease after stem cell transplantation can lead to vaginal dryness, adhesions, fibrosis, stenosis and vaginal shortening, resulting in pain and an inability to have penetrative sex. Breast surgery may cause altered appearance and breast sensation, while vulval surgery can result in introital stenosis or reduced clitoral sensitivity that leads to sexual pain or orgasmic changes.

In men, erectile dysfunction may result from hormonal changes secondary to androgen deprivation therapy, or result from nerve damage and vascular changes following pelvic surgery or radiotherapy. Reduced orgasmic intensity, dry or retrograde ejaculation and climacturia after pelvic surgery or radiotherapy also have a negative impact on men's sexual expression following cancer treatment.[3]

Anxiety and depression, body image adjustment, altered femininity or masculinity, infertility concerns, relationship strain and broader social difficulties are also common precipitating and maintaining factors for sexual difficulties associated with cancer.

Clinical assessment

In the oncology follow-up clinic, discussion of disease surveillance and acute side effects is generally prioritized over the assessment and management of late effects of treatment. Discussing the sexual consequences of cancer remains a challenging aspect of communication for health professionals and patients alike:[4] such conversations are more likely to be reported by male (68%) than by female (43%) cancer patients,[5] perhaps reflecting the greater number of biomedical treatments available for the management of erectile dysfunction.[6]

The increased use of brief clinical screeners and patient-reported outcome measures (PROMs) (Table 14.1) may assist busy clinicians to introduce and structure clinical discussions around sensitive topics such as sexual morbidity. Screening instruments are particularly helpful in settings where problem identification and onward referral for specialist assessment and treatment are anticipated. Detailed PROMs to evaluate sexual morbidity are more useful when management expertise is immediately available. However, reliance upon screening tools and checklists should not thwart appropriate discussions of people's sexual concerns, or reduce clinical discussion to a 'tick box' exercise.

The aim of assessment is to integrate biopsychosocial information to reach a tentative categorization or formulation of the individual's or couple's sexual difficulty. One simple formulation structure is the '5 Ps': presenting problem, precipitating factors, perpetuating factors, predisposing factors and protective factors.

Integrated management of treatment-associated sexual difficulties

The most common sexual consequences encountered in people affected by cancer are as follows:

- Loss of sexual interest.
- Male and female arousal difficulties.
- Sexual pain.
- Orgasmic and ejaculatory difficulties.

Sexual inactivity after cancer treatment is not problematic when the person is not dissatisfied, distressed or avoiding sex because of difficulties.

Table 14.1 Examples of clinical screeners for sexual concerns or difficulties.

Screener	Clinical utility
IIEF-5 or SHIM	• Five validated items extracted from 15-item IIEF • Likert response options • Rapid completion time • Assesses severity of erectile dysfunction • Does not evaluate desire, ejaculatory or orgasmic changes • Research and clinical use in oncology (mainly urology)
FSFI-6	• Six validated items extracted from 19-item FSFI • Likert response options • Rapid completion time • Assesses desire, subjective arousal, vaginal lubrication, orgasm, sexual satisfaction and sexual pain • Not yet validated for use in oncology
Single-item checklist screener for sexual concerns/problems in men and women, developed by Flynn et al.[7]	• Checklist screener identifies common male and female sexual difficulties • Patient checks all statements that apply • Rapid completion time • Not yet validated specifically for use in oncology

FSFI, Female Sexual Function Index; IIEF, International Index of Erectile Function; SHIM, Sexual Health Inventory for Men.

Optimal management of sexual difficulties is often achieved through judicious integration of biomedical, psychological and relationship strategies (Table 14.2). Psychological therapy may be appropriate where anxiety or low mood, altered body image, masculinity/femininity, infertility concerns or relationship difficulties are contributing to loss of sexual interest. Sexual desire often returns as the person recovers physically from initial treatment, or when high anxiety and low mood have improved. However, unremitting low desire commonly accompanies endocrine treatment for breast or prostate cancer and may be a source of distress, or make treatment compliance difficult over time. In these circumstances, psychosexual therapy may be helpful in reducing individual/couple distress and in enabling adaptation to altered patterns of desire, sexual responsiveness and expression.

Organic erectile dysfunction is frequently managed pharmacologically, although the response to drug therapy is variable and is usually dependent on the following:

- Patient and partner age (older age is associated with erectile dysfunction).

- Pretreatment erectile function.

- Presence of comorbidities (cardiovascular disease and diabetes are associated with a higher risk of erectile dysfunction).

- Nerve-sparing surgery (whether unilateral/bilateral or not).

Psychosexual therapy can be a useful adjunct to biomedical erectile dysfunction management, particularly when the response to drug treatment is limited and a poor response results from couple or individual factors amenable to therapy.[2,6] Psychosexual therapy is also appropriate in the management of more complex situations such as multiple physical comorbidities, sexual difficulties affecting both partners, or pre-existing sexual vulnerabilities exacerbated by cancer treatment, e.g. sexual abuse/violence, sexual fear/aversion or sexual pain.

Effective sexual pain management (Table 14.2) uses a combination of vaginal health strategies, pain management, physical therapy techniques and psychosexual therapy to address changes in vaginal dimensions, mucosal integrity and the woman's or couple's emotional and behavioural responses. Therapists often use a framework of behavioural exercises, called sensate focus, to break sexual expression down into smaller, manageable steps that assist gradual reintroduction of sensual contact, desensitization to painful stimuli, and progress towards vaginal penetration where feasible and desirable to the woman or couple.[2]

Adaptation to irreversible sexual changes

Some people's sexual difficulties are partially or not improved following biomedical and psychosocial interventions. These individuals or couples are likely to experience distress, and a common coping strategy is to avoid sexual intimacy. Avoidance of sexual intimacy can, however, disconnect people from a meaningful sexual relationship. Psychological and psychosexual therapy can facilitate the process of adjustment to the 'new normal'.

Third-wave cognitive behavioural therapies, such as acceptance and commitment therapy,[8] are particularly suited to helping people adjust to their altered sexual functioning and its psychosexual sequelae. Acceptance and commitment therapy aims to increase psychological flexibility by teaching people the skills to open up to distressing thoughts, emotions and sensations, rather than to experientially avoid them. Concurrently, people are supported to clarify what is important to them in their sexual relationship(s), as values are a helpful anchor in guiding and motivating behaviour. For example, a man has had a penile implant following prostate cancer but is

Table 14.2 Integrated management of sexual consequences of treatment.

Management	Loss of sexual interest	Arousal difficulties (objective/subjective)	Sexual pain	Orgasmic and ejaculatory changes
Biomedical	*Women* Endocrine review • Systemic HRT ± testosterone and/or vaginal oestrogen* *Men* Endocrine review • Testosterone supplementation* • Review/revise if likely medication side effect (e.g. antidepressants)	*Women* Vaginal dryness • Lubricants, vaginal moisturizers, topical oestrogen, systemic HRT* *Men* Erectile dysfunction • Oral phosphodiesterase type 5 inhibitors • Topical alprostadil (intraurethral pellet, ointment or intracavernosal injection) • Vacuum erection device • Testosterone supplementation* • Penile constriction rings/loops • Surgically placed penile implants	*Women* Gynaecology/women's health review • HRT/vaginal oestrogen* • Non-hormonal vaginal moisturizers • Vaginal lubricants (water-, oil- or silicone-based) • Vaginal dilators Pain clinic • Topical/systemic analgesia Physiotherapy • Pelvic floor assessment • Kegel exercises • Biofeedback *Men* (genital pain uncommon) Urology/andrology review • Urethral dilation (stricture) • Antibiotics (prostatitis) Analgesics for ejaculatory or neuropathic pain • Topical/systemic analgesia, e.g. NSAIDs and/or neuropathic pain agents	*Men* Urology/andrology review • Alpha agonist, e.g. ephedrine for retrograde ejaculation • Analgesia, e.g. NSAIDs and/or neuropathic pain agents for ejaculatory pain

Psychological therapy	Address anxiety/relaxation techniques/depression/review antidepressant medication effects/body image/femininity/masculinity/infertility concerns/identify sexual and relationship values, couple communication training
Psycho-education	Causation of organic/psychogenic sexual difficulties
	Barriers/enablers of sexual interest, adequate arousal and orgasmic release
	Subjective and objective arousal (erection or vaginal lubrication) mechanisms (arousal circuit)
	Fight–flight response
	Orgasm/ejaculation differentiation
	Pelvic floor rehabilitation, voiding prior to sex/condom use (climacturia post-prostatectomy)
Psychosexual therapy	Sensate focus/mindfulness to explore diverse/alternative sources of desire/arousal/climax
	De/reconstruct beliefs on definition of 'sex'
	Erotic fantasy, literature/images for arousal/orgasmic difficulties
	Wax and wane masturbatory exercises (male arousal difficulties), mindful masturbatory exercises, vibratory stimulation
	Vaginal desensitization–digital exploration, dilators, vibrators (female sexual pain)
	Penile/genital desensitization through structured touch/massage (male sexual pain)

*Seek advice from treating clinician regarding oncological safety before prescribing HRT or testosterone in oestrogen-driven tumours, or testosterone after prostate cancer treatment

HRT, hormone replacement therapy; NSAIDs, non-steroidal anti-inflammatory drugs.

embarrassed to use it and is therefore avoiding sexual activity with his partner, which has an unhelpful effect on their relationship. His therapist may guide him to do the following:

- Recognize what the embarrassment (emotion) feels like in his body (sensation) and teach him the skills to tolerate, regulate and validate (acceptance) it.
- Identify thoughts that contribute to the embarrassment, such as 'this should happen naturally, it's so clumsy'. Subsequently, he would be taught to 'unhook' from the thought so that he can look 'at' it rather than 'through' it, as this perspective reduces the impact of the thought.
- Clarify what qualities are important for him to bring to his sexual relationship (e.g. initiation, fun, passion) and to consider whether his current sexual avoidance takes him closer to or further away from these values.

Therapy often explores and encourages new definitions of 'sex' to enable someone to see themselves as a sexual person again, as this has a positive impact on their view of themselves and their relationship(s). For example, a woman with sexual pain, who struggles to have penetrative sex, may be more likely to recover her sexual desire and be more satisfied with her sex life if she subscribes to the belief that 'sex' is not solely defined by penetration, but by a range of sexual behaviours. Clinical experience suggests that men struggle more than women to shift from a narrower to a broader definition of sex.

Couples with a secure bond perceive each other as accessible, responsive and emotionally engaged and therefore find it easier to approach each other about difficulties.[9] The more secure their relationship, the better able they will be to face the illness/treatment-associated assaults on their sexual relationship. Conversely, couples whose relationship bond is insecure are more likely to pursue or withdraw in response to distress and are less likely to manage sexual difficulties on their own. These couples may benefit from a referral for relationship therapy prior to or integrated with sex therapy.

Conclusion

The management of cancer-related sexual difficulties requires a biopsychosocial framework, with a particular emphasis on psychosexual adaptation and flexibility. More robust evidence for the effectiveness and feasibility of psychosexual interventions should lead to increased uptake of integrated biopsychosocial management to improve care quality and outcomes.[10,11]

Further developments in survivorship practice and service provision are necessary if identification and management of treatment-induced sexual difficulties are to be improved in oncology. Training in communication and routine clinical assessment of sexual morbidity, development of local clinical guidelines and greater awareness of national organizations and services in sexual medicine and psychosexual therapy are all strategies that can enhance professional confidence and competence in this challenging facet of cancer rehabilitation.[2]

References

1 Mitchell KR, Mercer MH, Ploubidis GB, *et al.* Sexual function in Britain: findings from the third National Survey of Sexual Attitudes and Lifestyles (Natsal-3). *Lancet* 2013; 382: 1817–29.

2 Reisman Y, Gianotten WL, eds. *Cancer, intimacy and sexuality: a practical approach.* Cham, Switzerland: Springer, 2017; 1–4.

3 Schover LR, van der Kaaij M, van Dorst E, *et al.* Sexual dysfunction and infertility as late effects of cancer treatment. *EJC Suppl* 2014; 12: 41–53.

4 White ID, Allan H, Faithfull S. Assessment of treatment-induced female sexual morbidity in oncology: is this a part of routine medical follow-up after radical pelvic radiotherapy? *Br J Cancer* 2011; 105: 903–10.

5 Gilbert E, Pertz J, Ussher JM. Talking about sex with health professionals: the experience of people with cancer and their partners. *Eur J Cancer Care (Engl)* 2016; 25: 280–93.

6 Kirby MG, White ID, Butcher J, *et al.* Development of UK recommendations on treatment for post-surgical erectile dysfunction. *Int J Clin Pract* 2014; 68: 590–608.

7 Flynn KE, Lindau ST, Lin L, *et al.* Development and validation of a single-item screener for self-reporting sexual problems in U.S. adults. *J Gen Intern Med* 2015; 30: 1468–75.

8 Hayes SC, Strosahl KD, Wilson KG. *Acceptance and commitment therapy. The process and practice of mindful change.* London: Guildford Press, 2011.

9 Johnson S, Zuccarini D. Integrating sex and attachment in emotionally focused couple therapy. *J Marit Family Ther* 2009; 46: 431–45.

10 Brotto LA, Yule M, Breckon E. Psychological interventions for the sexual sequelae of cancer. *J Cancer Surviv* 2010; 4: 346–60.

11 Kim J-H, Yang Y, Hwang E-S. The effectiveness of psychoeducational interventions focused on sexuality in cancer. *Cancer Nurs* 2015; 38: E32–42.

15 Social Difficulties of Cancer Patients

Penny Wright, Peter Selby

Introduction

Cancer represents a substantial burden on individuals, society and the economy. Traditionally an approach to cancer patients focused on accurate diagnosis and treatment interventions aimed to maximize survival. Elsewhere in this book we describe the move towards patient-centred care, which includes recognition of the need to measure and prioritize the psychological aspects of the patient's experience and to put in place effective supportive measures. In this chapter we review progress towards identifying and measuring the social difficulties of cancer patients and indicate the available measures to address these.

The social impact of cancer

The social impact of cancer may be considerable not only at the time of diagnosis, when immediate readjustments may have to be made, but also possibly over many years following diagnosis. Some cancer 'survivors' will be disease-free following their treatment, but others may attend hospital for monitoring, for multiple treatment cycles for chronic cancer[1] or for palliative interventions.[2] Side and late effects of treatment are not uncommon, which may result in chronic disability and restrictions in carrying out daily activities. Patients at all stages of disease report problems in all domains of life.[3]

- In the home (e.g. domestic chores, personal care, caring responsibilities).
- With services (e.g. support services, aids and adaptations).
- With finances (e.g. welfare benefits, mortgages/pensions), and regarding employment.
- Legally (e.g. sorting out family affairs, wills).
- With relationships (e.g. communication problems, new relationships).
- Concerning sexuality and body image, as well as recreationally (e.g. social and leisure activities, holidays).
- With housing and getting around.

In addition to the direct impact of cancer and cancer treatment on everyday living, there are indirect 'knock-on' effects. For example, a patient may experience financial difficulties as a result of cancer and its treatment (e.g. loss of income or increased daily living costs), leading to detrimental impacts on family life, roles and relationships.[4] A qualitative study found that patients and carers reported being unprepared for the financial impact following a cancer diagnosis, delaying taking action to address financial problems, which in some cases led to significant long-term problems such as debt or house repossession.[4] The impact of cancer on employment and family economics can be profound.[5,6] Timmons *et al.*[6] stated: 'This study reveals the complex, multidimensional nature of the financial and economic burden cancer imposes on patients and the whole family unit. Changes in income after cancer exacerbate the effects of cancer-related out-of-pocket expenses. These findings have implications for healthcare professionals, service providers and policy makers.'

Who is at risk?

Although most patients are resilient and cope with the impact of cancer and its treatment on their lives, a significant minority struggle. In a population-based survey of more than 17,000 colorectal cancer patients,[7] 15% of participants reported levels of social distress (measured using the 21-item Social Difficulties Inventory [SDI-21]) which if found in clinical practice would have warranted some form of further assessment or discussion with the clinical team. Clinical and treatment-related factors, including advanced disease and having a stoma, and pre-existing sociodemographic characteristics were associated with poorer social outcomes. This held true across all 'social' domains (at home, at work, at leisure, in relationships); age (under 55 or over 85), having multiple comorbidities, unemployment and having caring responsibilities were strong independent predictors of poor outcome across all domains of everyday life.[7]

Assessment of social difficulties

The existence of social problems has been well recognized over recent decades, and there is a growing body of evidence on prevalence and intensity. Social problems may contribute to multiple, chronic problems and poorer mental health. Patients with multiple concerns or difficulties, including social problems, have been shown to be more likely to exhibit clinically significant anxiety or depression.[8] Therefore, early detection by clinical teams and intervention by support services might be appropriate in some cases. How to provide relevant supportive care for those who need it in a timely, cost-effective way is, however, a challenge. In 2007 the National Cancer Survivorship Initiative was launched jointly with the Department of Health and Macmillan Cancer Support. It included introduction of a structured holistic needs assessment and provision of a care plan, followed in 2013 with models for providing support including the introduction of health and well-being clinics.[2] Although progress has been made in regard to fulfilling these recommendations, there is still much to be done. In 2015 only 33% of patients responding to the National Cancer Patient Experience Survey had been given a care plan. Information provision from staff concerning finance and work was varied.[9]

In Canada, the Distress Assessment and Response Tool (DART) programme provides an efficient and effective way of identifying those most at risk of poor social outcomes, leading to provision of appropriate advice, signposting for supportive self-management and referral to services for those most in need.[10] Hospital-wide DART screening has been sustained at 70% for the last 3 years. One of the key strategies for successful implementation was to use a multi-symptom tool rather than only screening for emotional distress.

SDI-21

One of the measures incorporated in the DART assessment is the SDI-21. This is one of a number of instruments designed to assess social problems. Unlike some measures, the SDI-21 has been well reviewed and covers a number of social domains rather than focusing on just one area such as finances.[11,12] The SDI-21 fulfils requirements of brevity, simplicity, relevance, and flagging problems of practical significance for use in screening in routine practice.[13] It comprises 21 questions about various everyday worries commonly experienced by cancer patients, answered on a scale of 0 'no difficulty' to 3 'very much difficulty', with respect to the previous month, such that higher scores are indicative of greater social problems. The scale has good psychometric properties and a clear factor structure. Sixteen of the items form an interval scale of social distress (SD-16), which comprises three subscales: everyday living, money matters, and self and others.[14] A clinically meaningful scoring system is able to identify a significant number of patients requiring information or referral to specialist services.[15,16] Preliminary analysis indicates that the SD-16 can predict longer term health-related quality-of-life outcomes among cancer survivors[17] and is being used not only for individual patient screening but also in research and in large-scale population cancer patient-reported outcome surveys in colorectal, bladder, prostate, and head and neck cancer.

Conclusion

 Implementing a programme such as DART is a gold standard for identifying and providing appropriate intervention for those in need. It has been developed using a bottom-up and top-down process so that all staff value the programme. It is reliant on a well-supported electronic platform for administration, scoring and reporting the assessment and subsequent supportive care interventions. Most hospitals in the UK do not have access to such systems, although over time they are likely to become more commonplace. So what options are available now to cancer clinical teams to spot those patients who are socially distressed and provide them with the support they need?

Top tips

- If you have an electronic assessment system, start using it and encourage others to do so too.

- If possible, use a screening tool for assessment that has clear clinical guidance on how scores may be interpreted.

- If you do not have access to a simple screening process, keep in mind those patients who may be most at risk of social distress:
  - those with advanced disease (chronic cancer and palliative care patients);
  - those with side and late effects of treatment (e.g. stoma, pelvic radiation disease, lymphoedema);
  - those with comorbidity (e.g. diabetes, mental health problems, arthritis);
  - those of pre-retirement age;
  - those who are frail or very elderly;
  - those who are unemployed;
  - those who have caring responsibilities (e.g. frail, dependent partner, or children).

- You cannot be all things to all patients; therefore, have available up-to-date information about:
  - where patients may go to get good information for self-management (e.g. websites, leaflets, support groups);
  - available services for different types of problem identified for referral (e.g. social services, psychology, physiotherapy).

- Some patients at low risk of cancer recurrence but with complex problems may be better managed by key generalists (e.g. GP, care of the elderly team, community social care).

- Do not be frightened of asking patients how they are managing in their everyday lives. Remember that most people are resilient and prefer to cope using resources available to them (e.g. family, friends, employers, financial advisers): picking something up sooner may prevent more complex problems arising later.

- A good intervention is a simple acknowledgement from you that it is hard to cope with cancer. Many patients feel better just knowing that others recognize their difficulties and that what they are experiencing is not unusual.

- Record what you have discussed and pass this on to relevant colleagues (e.g. GP, clinical nurse specialist, other specialists). This will help with continuity of care and avoid duplication of effort.

References

1 Harley C, Pini S, Bartlett YK, Velikova G. Defining chronic cancer: patient experiences and self-management needs. *BMJ Support Palliat Care* 2015; 5: 343–50.

2 Department of Health, Macmillan Cancer Support, NHS Improvement. *Living with and beyond cancer: taking action to improve outcomes (an update to the 2010 the National Cancer Survivorship Initiative vision)*. London: Department of Health, 2013.

3 Wright EP, Kiely MA, Lynch P, *et al.* Social problems in oncology. *Br J Cancer* 2002; 87: 1099–104.

4 Amir Z, Wilson K, Hennings J, Young A. The meaning of cancer: implications for family finances and consequent impact on lifestyle, activities, roles and relationships. *Psychooncology* 2012; 21: 1167–74.

5 Paalman CH, van Leeuwen FE, Aaronson NK, *et al.* Employment and social benefits up to 10 years after breast cancer diagnosis: a population-based study. *Br J Cancer* 2016; 114: 81–7.

6 Timmons A, Gooberman-Hill R, Sharp L. The multidimensional nature of the financial and economic burden of a cancer diagnosis on patients and their families: qualitative findings from a country with a mixed public–private healthcare system. *Support Care Cancer* 2013; 21: 107–17.

7 Wright P, Downing A, Morris EJA, *et al.* Identifying social distress: a cross-sectional survey of social outcomes 12 to 36 months after colorectal cancer diagnosis. *J Clin Oncol* 2015; 33: 3423–30.

8 Cull A, Stewart M, Altman DG. Assessment of and intervention for psychosocial problems in routine oncology practice. *Br J Cancer* 1995; 72: 229–35.

9 Quality Health (2016). *National Cancer Patient Experience Survey. 2015 National results summary*. Available from: www.ncpes.co.uk/index.php/reports/national-reports (accessed 8 February 2017).

10 Li M, Macedo A, Crawford S, *et al.* Easier said than done: keys to successful implementation of the Distress Assessment and Response Tool (DART) program. *J Oncol Pract* 2016; 12: e513–26.

11 Catt S, Starkings R, Shilling V, Fallowfield L. Patient-reported outcome measures of the impact of cancer on patients' everyday lives: a systematic review. *J Cancer Surviv* 2017; 11: 211–32.

12 Muzzatti B, Annunziata MA. Assessing the social impact of cancer: a review of available tools. *Support Care Cancer* 2012; 20: 2249–57.

13 Wright EP, Kiely M, Johnston C, *et al.* Development and evaluation of an instrument to assess social difficulties in routine oncology practice. *Qual Life Res* 2005; 14: 373–86.

14 Wright P, Smith AB, Keding A, Velikova G. The Social Difficulties Inventory (SDI): development of subscales and scoring guidance for staff. *Psychooncology* 2011; 20: 36–43.

15 Wright P, Smith A, Roberts K, *et al.* Screening for social difficulties in cancer patients: clinical utility of the Social Difficulties Inventory. *Br J Cancer* 2007; 97: 1063–70.

16 Wright P, Marshall L, Smith A, *et al.* Measurement and interpretation of social distress using the Social Difficulties Inventory (SDI). *Eur J Cancer* 2008; 44: 1529–35.

17 Ashley L, Velikova G, Downing A, *et al.* Health-related quality of life in cancer survivorship: predictive power of the Social Difficulties Inventory. *Psychooncology* doi: 10.1002/pon.4368.

16 Complementary Therapies in Patient-Centred and Integrated Cancer Care

Jacqui Stringer

Introduction

The term 'complementary therapy' in cancer care is an amorphous one and has historically been identified with many different aspects of care, from nutritional supplements through to exercise, with many forms of intervention such as massage coming under the same umbrella. This, combined with the fact that until relatively recently the majority of such treatments were performed by non-healthcare professionals, has made it notoriously difficult to collate strong evidence of safety and efficacy for the myriad therapies available, and for clinicians to make informed choices as to whether to support such practice in relation to their own patients. To make the situation even more complex, until recently complementary therapies were always tied in with 'alternative' therapies: when patients chose not to continue with conventional medicine but instead try alternative routes to health. There are several therapies (e.g. nutrition, such as the Gerson diet, or herbal medicine) that can be used as a complement or alternative to conventional care. In order to make complementary therapies more acceptable in mainstream care, institutions have developed a variety of different terminologies to try and better express how therapies can support the care of the cancer patient, such as integrative therapies, complementary medicine and holistic therapies.

Many cancer centres and units either provide or have access to complementary therapies for their patients as a supportive measure to help relieve stress and facilitate a better quality of life during treatment. These are usually free and often charity-funded for NHS patients. The evolution of such services has occurred despite a lack of high-quality, peer-reviewed data and continues to develop, becoming almost an expectation, because of patient demand and staff observation of the perceived benefits. Cancer Research UK, for example, has a page on its website providing information for patients on how they can access therapies.

For clarity, this chapter is a reflection on the potential benefits of incorporating complementary therapies into mainstream healthcare for patients with cancer and their families. It is beyond the remit of this chapter to explore all complementary therapies offered in the cancer care setting; therefore, the focus is to show a spread of therapies used for different indications and suggest their potential for integration.

Acupuncture

Acupuncture is a complementary therapy with one of the largest evidence bases in oncology and related fields. A study by Molassiotis et al.[1] showed it to be a promising management technique for cancer-related fatigue, which is a significant cause of morbidity in this patient population. One of the challenges with acupuncture is the necessity for a series of weekly treatments (individual protocols may vary), with the usual course being 6 weeks and often with maintenance 'top-ups' to sustain symptomatic improvement. This can lead to issues around funding and additional visits. However, in the Molassiotis et al. study,[1] self-needling was successfully taught to participants and may provide a practical solution to long-term symptom control. In cases of problematic and complex symptoms, acupuncture is a useful tool, as core/standard points for the primary issue (e.g. pain) can be supplemented by additional points for secondary issues (e.g. poor sleep, anxiety, nausea) at the therapist's discretion. A current study funded by the National Institute for Health Research (A Trial of Acupuncture for People with Nerve Damage Symptoms Caused by Chemotherapy [ACUFOCIN]) is exploring the efficacy of using acupuncture as a management tool for chemotherapy-induced peripheral neuropathy, and the protocol has been developed to validate this way of working. What has yet to be explored is the cost-effectiveness of using acupuncture in mainstream services; there will be preliminary data relating to this from the above study, and a comprehensive assessment is planned if the results are positive.

In summary, while acupuncture is an invasive complementary therapy, there is a large and growing evidence base to validate its safety and efficacy in hard-to-manage symptoms. Additionally, regarding patient safety, many practitioners are also healthcare providers with a clear understanding of the possible issues related to working with this patient population.

Aromatherapy

This complementary therapy is based on the use of essential oils. Essential oils are volatile oils produced by the plant which gives the oil its name. They are complex compounds sometimes containing hundreds of chemical components. In the UK they are primarily used in holistic treatments (e.g. in addition to massage) and are non-toxic when used by a qualified practitioner in low concentrations. It is suggested that benefits experienced are primarily through the olfactory system, where they trigger feelings of, for example, relaxation, through their almost instant access to the limbic system. Audits into the use of essential oils through inhalation appear to validate this rationale.[2,3] In other countries (e.g. France), however, the primary mode of use is as a medicine, and education into prescribing essential oils is part of medical training. It is notoriously difficult to carry out clinical trials into the efficacy of using essential oils in the clinical field, as they contain multiple active ingredients and legislation is not set up to work with such compounds. There is, however, a growing body of literature from both laboratory and animal experiments validating some of the clinical benefits described in historical literature,[4] including the antimicrobial activity of many oils. Unpublished work from the University of Manchester (P. Warn. Personal communication, 2004) also indicates that certain oils work in synergy when blended and used with standard antimicrobial agents. Interestingly, the action of the oils tested did not appear to be affected by the presence of proteins. These data would suggest that they are ideal topical antimicrobials to use alongside standard treatments in complex, or infected, chronic wounds.[5] For the full benefits of essential oils to be harnessed much research is still required; however, awareness of their potential is starting to be recognized. This can be challenging, as the media occasionally publish poorly tested claims that certain oils, e.g. frankincense, can 'cure' cancer, thus prompting vulnerable people to start taking the oil in an uncontrolled and potentially toxic manner. It is to be hoped that funding can be acquired to develop the clinical use of these powerful and potentially very useful agents in a safe and methodical way.

Massage

Touch therapies are acknowledged to be some of the least invasive and easiest to provide complementary therapies in cancer care. The theory behind the perceived benefits of touch is based on psychoneuroimmunology.[6] Tiffany Field and her team at the Touch Research Institute in Miami have produced data over recent decades looking at the use of touch in different patient populations (e.g. preterm babies) and have consistently shown it to provide benefits such as reduction in stress, anxiety and stress hormone levels, and improvement in immune function.[7] As such, it is probably the least contentious complementary therapy to provide and can be used to facilitate reduction in anxiety and distress, help sleep and provide distraction from current circumstances.[8] It is, however, imperative that the practitioner is fully cognisant with contraindications in this patient population. Shorter sessions (e.g. 20 min) are often to be recommended and are sufficient to provide the benefits described without risk of the touch becoming an irritant.[8]

Reflexology is a form of touch therapy working peripheral parts of the body, usually the feet, based on the theory that points on the feet relate to corresponding areas of the body. In oncology it is used as a gentle foot massage, usually to aid relaxation, although improvements in symptoms such as pain are reported anecdotally.

Relaxation, creative visualization and stress management techniques

Helping patients and their families cope with the stresses associated with a diagnosis of cancer is one of the key aims of complementary therapies. Teaching them skills they can use when a therapist is not available is an important aspect of this. Teaching techniques for relaxation and visualizing a 'safe space' somewhere away from the hospital during an invasive procedure such as cannulation, for example, has been seen to be an effective method of managing anxiety. Hypnotherapy is a more intense technique for inducing relaxation and minimizing states of acute anxiety or panic and for managing phobias, and as such can be used for patients struggling to comply with treatment or scans (e.g. patients with head and neck tumours undergoing radiotherapy) due to feelings of claustrophobia.[9] Using such techniques can not only enhance the patient experience but can also reduce the amount of medication, additional staff time and treatment delays associated with managing such situations. It is not a risk-free technique, as the 'scripts' used to induce relaxation or trance have to be acceptable to the patient or they can have a negative effect. It is therefore important for the practitioner to be experienced with working in the field of oncology and to be aware of what cancer treatments entail as well as patients' own preferences.[10] That said, these complementary therapies show much promise in managing anxiety and may be used to screen patients for underlying mental health issues which may require more specialist interventions. In-house evaluation of the service provided at The Christie NHS Foundation Trust using the Hospital Anxiety and Depression Scale before and after intervention has provided preliminary validation of this way of working. Further research is under development.

Conclusion

It is beyond the remit of this chapter to explore all complementary therapies available; therefore, only some of those seen as having most benefit, associated literature and promise for integration into standard care have been highlighted. They have also been chosen to give readers some clarity on how similar complementary therapies may be of use. Mindfulness, for example, has not been discussed specifically but is a technique of use in helping patients stay focused rather than becoming overwhelmed by intrusive, negative thoughts; as such it is a different but related method of managing stress. It is worth noting that these complementary therapies can be used in combination to achieve maximum effect through multiple sensory input.

References

1 Molassiotis A, Bardy J, Finnegan-John J, *et al.* Acupuncture for cancer-related fatigue in patients with breast cancer: a pragmatic randomized controlled trial. *J Clin Oncol* 2012; 30: 4470–6.

2 Dyer J, Cleary L, Ragsdale-Lowe M, *et al.* The use of aromasticks in a cancer centre: a retrospective audit. *Complement Ther Clin Pract* 2014; 20: 2013–206.

3 Dyer J, Cleary L, McNeill S, *et al.* The use of aromasticks to help with sleep problems: a patient experience survey. *Complement Ther Clin Pract* 2016; 22: 51–8.

4 Buckle J. *Clinical aromatherapy: essential oils in healthcare.* 3rd ed. St Louis, MO: Elsevier, 2015.

5 Stringer J, Donald G, Knowles R, Warn P. The symptom management of fungating malignant wounds using a novel essential oil cream. *Wounds UK* 2014; 10: 30–8.

6 Field T. *Touch.* 2nd ed. Cambridge, MA: MIT Press, 2003.

7 Hernandez-Reif M, Ironson G, Field T, *et al.* Breast cancer patients have improved immune and neuroendocrine functions following massage therapy. *J Psychosom Res* 2004; 57: 45–52.

8 Stringer J, Swindell R, Dennis M. Massage in patients undergoing intensive chemotherapy reduces serum cortisol and prolactin. *Psychooncology* 2008; 17: 1024–31.

9 Mackereth PA, Tomlinson L, Maycock P, *et al.* Calming panic states in the mould room and beyond: a pilot complementary therapy head and neck cancer service. *J Radiother Pract* 2012; 11: 83–91.

10 Carter A, Mackereth PA. *Aromatherapy, massage and relaxation in cancer care: an integrative resource for practitioners.* London: Singing Dragon, 2017.

17 Fertility Issues in Cancer Treatment

Rebecca Lee, Anne Armstrong

Introduction

Approximately 10% of newly diagnosed cancers in the UK occur in individuals aged between 15 and 49 years.[1] Owing to the increase in cancer incidence with age, the trend towards delayed childbirth means that there is a higher chance of being diagnosed with cancer before families are complete. In 2015, over half (53%) of all live births in England and Wales were to mothers aged 30 and over, and two-thirds (68%) of fathers were aged 30 and over.[2] Furthermore, improvements in treating cancer have resulted in greater numbers of survivors for whom fertility is an important issue.

Many cancer treatments can affect fertility, either directly through gynaecological surgery or through targeting of rapidly dividing cells by systemic therapies, affecting the reproductive organs and endocrine system.[3] The effects of surgery, chemotherapy and radiotherapy on reproductive function have been the most extensively documented; however, other treatments can have direct or indirect effects on fertility. Chemotherapy and radiotherapy can cause temporary, long-term or permanent reduction in sperm counts. Radiation and alkylating agents are most likely to cause long-term or permanent azoospermia.[4] Recovery of sperm production depends on the survival of spermatogonial stem cells and can take years. It is therefore important to counsel patients that fertility can recover eventually and therefore contraception should still be considered.

Radiation can also affect female reproduction in a variety of ways, either by disrupting the functioning of the hypothalamic–pituitary axis, causing ovarian failure, or causing damage to the uterus that prevents gestation of a fetus to full term.[3] Chemotherapy causes direct toxicity to the ovaries and may cause permanent or temporary cessation of menses.[3] The risk of amenorrhoea varies according to the chemotherapy regimen used and the woman's age at treatment. To complicate matters further, treatments such as tamoxifen, while not adversely affecting fertility, are teratogenic and are therefore contraindicated during pregnancy and prior to conception. During the extended 5–10 years of tamoxifen therapy a woman's fertility is likely to decline significantly.

Many national and international guidelines have been created which advise on the implications and management of fertility issues in patients with cancer.[3-6] Most of the guidance, however, is based on cohort and case–control studies due to the lack of randomized evidence in this area. This chapter will focus on how fertility concerns affect patients with cancer and how physicians can improve the assessment, discussion and management of fertility issues in patients undergoing cancer therapy.

Importance of fertility to patients

While survival from cancer is a priority, fertility issues have been shown to be hugely important for cancer patients.[7] Increased concerns about fertility have been correlated with increased psychological morbidity.[8] One study of 131 women with early-stage breast cancer showed that recalled reproductive concerns were an independent predictor of consistent depressive symptoms ($p=0.04$).[8]

Many cancer survivors report concerns regarding fertility, both at diagnosis and following treatment. A web-based survey among 657 breast cancer survivors revealed that 57% recalled substantial concern at diagnosis about infertility associated with treatment.[9] A study examining attitudes to fertility in women with ovarian cancer showed that approximately 50% feared the cancer could affect their ability to reproduce.[10] A study among 96 young men newly diagnosed with cancer showed that having children ranked as their third highest priority (out of eight life goals), just behind good health and success at school or work.[11] Many studies have also reported that the quality of life (QOL) of adolescents can be affected by fertility concerns both at the time of diagnosis and following treatment.[12]

Furthermore, fertility issues have been shown to affect cancer therapy decisions made by patients. A prospective study of 620 patients with breast cancer revealed that 1% chose not to receive chemotherapy because of fertility-related concerns, 3% decided not to receive endocrine therapy, and 11% considered receiving endocrine therapy for less than 5 years.[13] A survey of young women with breast cancer reported that 29% admitted that infertility concerns influenced their treatment decisions.[9]

These findings emphasize the importance to patients of maintaining fertility and the need to incorporate fertility discussions into patient care.

Barriers to fertility discussions

Many barriers have been identified in discussing fertility issues with cancer patients.[7] They include physicians prioritizing treatment issues rather than QOL after treatment, lack of knowledge regarding fertility preservation techniques, and concerns over delays in treatment and increasing emotional distress. In adolescent cancer, initiating a dialogue with both the patient and the family can be an additional challenge.

Information needs

Studies have shown that patients report receiving inadequate fertility information.[7,14] Many papers have identified that patients need improved information regarding the risk of cancer treatments to fertility and the availability of fertility preservation options.[7] A questionnaire-based study in 228 women with breast cancer reported that patients had unmet needs for fertility-related information, and it highlighted the importance of revisiting fertility discussions during a patient's cancer treatment.[14]

Overview of fertility assessment and discussion

A guide to incorporating fertility discussions into patients' treatment pathway is provided in Figure 17.1. It is important to discuss fertility and preservation strategies in a timely manner to prevent delay to cancer therapy.[7] This is particularly critical for women, as egg preservation strategies can take a number of weeks depending on timing of the menstrual cycle. NICE guidelines recommend that the impact of cancer and its treatment on fertility should be discussed with patients at diagnosis and cryopreservation offered where appropriate.[6]

In assessing patients for assisted reproduction, it is important to take into account the diagnosis, treatment plan, expected outcome of fertility treatment, cancer prognosis and viability of stored sperm/gametes/embryos.[6] NICE guidelines state that the conventional eligibility criteria for infertility treatments in the UK do not apply to people with cancer, and infertility treatments should be offered to all patients of reproductive age.[6] In cases where delay to cancer treatment may

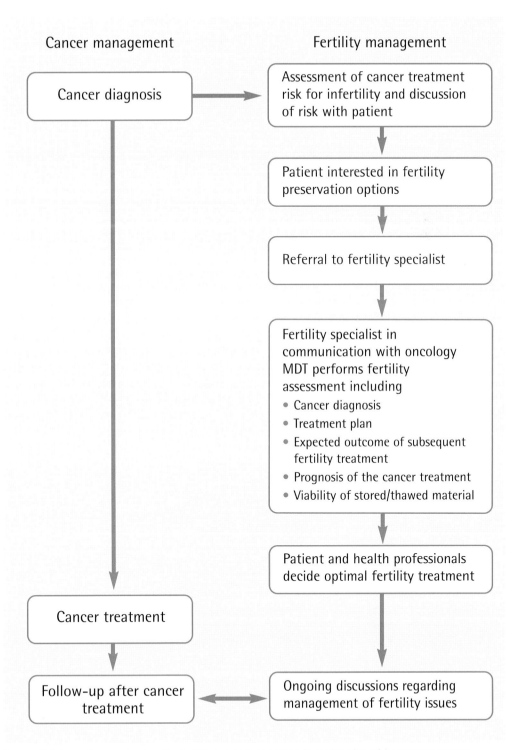

Figure 17.1 Flow diagram showing the fertility assessment process in conjunction with cancer treatment.

affect outcome, the risks should be explained so that patients can make informed decisions. One study showed that loss of choice surrounding fertility is particularly difficult for patients undergoing cancer treatment; therefore, involving them in the decision-making process is important, even if the outcome remains the same.[7] Tools are available to aid fertility-associated decision making in patients with cancer.[15] A study evaluating a decision aid in 120 women with breast cancer showed that patients using the tool had reduced decisional conflict after 1 year and were more satisfied with the fertility information provided compared with women receiving standard care.[15]

Finally, many studies have shown that referral to a fertility specialist is integral to the treatment pathway; therefore, a clear referral pathway should be incorporated into the multidisciplinary team (MDT) strategy.[7] MDT members should be identified who are responsible for ensuring fertility discussions take place and that referrals are made in a timely fashion. In order to achieve prioritization for fertility treatment, close working relationships need to be made with fertility specialists and clear protocols should be developed to incorporate fertility treatment into the pathway.

Recent developments

Improvements in fertility-sparing techniques in gynaecological cancers such as radical vaginal trachelectomy and ovarian transposition will continue to reduce the impact of surgery on fertility. Advances in assisted reproductive techniques are likely to increase fertility preservation options available to patients with cancer. Development of cryopreservation of testicular tissue is still experimental but will be an important step towards preserving fertility of prepubertal boys. Ovarian cryopreservation and subsequent autotransplantation is technically possible, and there have been reports of live births; however, there remains the risk of preserving and transplanting malignant cells.[5] More widely available, 'random start' stimulation protocols allow ovarian stimulation to start at any time during the menstrual cycle, reducing delays to cancer treatment.[5] Pharmacological protection of the ovaries using luteinizing hormone-releasing hormone analogues (LHRHa) during chemotherapy reduces rates of ovarian failure and may result in a greater number of pregnancies.[5] The mechanism by which LHRHa reduce gonadotoxicity is, however, not completely understood.

As our ability to predict ovarian reserve improves, we will be better able to counsel patients on the likely success, or otherwise, of conception. This is particularly relevant in patients on ongoing anticancer therapies such as tamoxifen, where a decision to interrupt active treatment may be influenced by the likelihood of conception. Such women are eligible for enrolment into the Pregnancy Outcome and Safety of Interrupting Therapy for Women with Endocrine-Responsive Breast Cancer (POSITIVE) study, which is collecting prospective data to understand the impact of interrupting tamoxifen in women with oestrogen receptor (ER)-positive breast cancer in order to conceive.

The potential impact of new agents on future fertility is rarely a priority for drug development, with most trials taking appropriate steps to ensure unexpected pregnancies on therapy do not occur. As agents move from the metastatic to the adjuvant setting, long-term impacts on fertility become more relevant. It is important that healthcare professionals keep up to date with studies investigating late effects from novel therapies and counsel patients accordingly.

Conclusion

Fertility issues are extremely important to patients and can affect their decisions about cancer treatment and their QOL after treatment. It is essential that fertility discussions take place early in the treatment pathway in order to initiate measures to preserve fertility without delay to cancer management.

References

1 Wilkes S, Coulson S, Crosland A, *et al.* Experience of fertility preservation among younger people diagnosed with cancer. *Hum Fertil* 2010; 13: 151–8.

2 Office for National Statistics (2016). *Births by parents' characteristics in England and Wales: 2015.* Available from: www.ons.gov.uk/peoplepopulationandcommunity/birthsdeathsandmarriages/livebirths/bulletins/birthsbyparentscharacteristicsinenglandandwales/2015 (accessed 12 March 2017).

3 Peccatori FA, Azim HA, Orecchia R, *et al.* Cancer, pregnancy and fertility: ESMO clinical practice guidelines for diagnosis, treatment and follow-up. *Ann Oncol* 2013; 24 (suppl 6): vi160–70.

4 American Society of Clinical Oncology. ASCO recommendations on fertility preservation in cancer patients: guideline summary. *J Oncol Pract* 2006; 2: 143–6.

5 Lambertini M, Del Mastro L, Pescio MC, *et al.* Cancer and fertility preservation: international recommendations from an expert meeting. *BMC Med* 2016; 14: 1.

6 National Institute for Health and Care Excellence (2013). *Fertility problems: assessment and treatment. Clinical guideline CG156.* Available from: www.nice.org.uk/guidance/CG156 (accessed 12 March 2017).

7 Lee RJ, Wakefield A, Foy S, *et al.* Facilitating reproductive choices: the impact of health services on the experiences of young women with breast cancer. *Psychooncology* 2011; 20: 1044–52.

8 Gorman JR, Malcarne VL, Roesch SC, *et al.* Depressive symptoms among young breast cancer survivors: the importance of reproductive concerns. *Breast Cancer Res Treat* 2010; 123: 477–85.

9 Partridge AH, Gelber S, Peppercorn J, *et al.* Web-based survey of fertility issues in young women with breast cancer. *J Clin Oncol* 2004; 22: 4174–83.

10 Zanagnolo V, Sartori E, Trussardi E, *et al.* Preservation of ovarian function, reproductive ability and emotional attitudes in patients with malignant ovarian tumors. *Eur J Obstet Gynecol Reprod Biol* 2005; 123: 235–43.

11 Klosky JL, Simmons JL, Russell KM, *et al.* Fertility as a priority among at-risk adolescent males newly diagnosed with cancer and their parents. *Support Care Cancer* 2015; 23: 333–41.

12 Nahata L, Quinn GP. Fertility preservation in young males at risk for infertility: what every pediatric provider should know. *J Adolesc Health* 2017; 60: 237–8.

13 Ruddy KJ, Gelber SI, Tamimi RM, *et al.* Prospective study of fertility concerns and preservation strategies in young women with breast cancer. *J Clin Oncol* 2014; 32: 1151–6.

14 Thewes B, Meiser B, Taylor A, *et al.* Fertility- and menopause-related information needs of younger women with a diagnosis of early breast cancer. *J Clin Oncol* 2005; 23: 5155–65.

15 Peate M, Meiser B, Cheah BC, *et al.* Making hard choices easier: a prospective, multicentre study to assess the efficacy of a fertility-related decision aid in young women with early-stage breast cancer. *Br J Cancer* 2012; 106: 1053–61.

18 Embedding Patient and Public Involvement and Engagement in a Cancer Research Centre

Jim Fitzgibbon, Kate Cleary, Annmarie Nelson

Background

The progress that has been made to develop patient-centred cancer care, and the important role that patient and public involvement and engagement (PPIE) have played, are described in this book. It is, however, acknowledged that these vital approaches are not fully embedded everywhere in the UK or internationally. In this chapter we explain the systematic efforts to embed PPIE in our cancer centres, the challenges we have met and the progress we have made, as a practical aid to others who are following this path. Our focus is on research, but our experience is usually relevant to service development and delivery.

The Wales Cancer Research Centre is funded by the Welsh Government and is a key part of its research infrastructure via Health and Care Research Wales. Led from Cardiff University, it has an all-Wales brief, with partners ranging across NHS Wales, Welsh universities, cancer charities and the pharmaceutical industry. The Wales Cancer Research Centre coordinates cancer research across four themes.

- Preclinical research supports laboratory studies that define the mechanisms of cancer development and progression, and identify potential diagnostics, biomarkers and treatments that can be used in clinical research settings to improve patient outcomes.

- Translational research brings discoveries from the laboratory bench to the bedside and from the bedside to the bench, in return.

- Clinical research involves implementing the findings of preclinical and translational research and is the first stage where new therapies are brought to patients to trial.

- Community research focuses on three areas of strategic importance in improving patient outcomes and experience: (1) screening, prevention and early diagnosis; (2) sharing of data; and (3) palliative and supportive care research.

We have been working towards best practice integration of PPIE across all of these diverse research areas.

The beginning of PPIE

When the Wales Cancer Research Centre was established in April 2015, there was discussion about whether PPIE should be a fifth theme, given the status that might imply, or should in some way encompass or infuse the four research themes. In the end it was decided that it should not be a separate entity alongside the four research themes, but should be seen as a 'golden thread' (the term used at the centre's launch) to be woven into everything the centre did. Other decisions taken at the earliest stage were as follows:

- To embed a lay perspective within an evaluated and rigorous framework; the 'thread' should be led collaboratively by a lay lead and an academic lead, establishing the PPIE function as one of partnership.

- To use the term 'research partner' to describe the role undertaken by lay people recruited to the project. It is a term long used in Wales in preference to other titles because it describes more precisely the willing coming together of researchers and lay people to undertake the best possible research.

- Each theme should have attached to it two research partners whose primary roles would be to facilitate and identify good PPIE practice and share it within the centre, agree with researchers gaps that hindered further progress, and take a lead in filling those gaps.

- PPIE should be represented in the centre's governance at both strategic and operational levels. As the research partners became well known they were invited to other tiers and types of meetings to gain input from them. Significantly, the lay lead, alongside the four theme leads and the centre director, is a member of the executive advisory board.

- A PPIE advisory group (later the word 'advisory' was dropped) was established to steer the development of policy and practice and the production of documents to support the themes. Those documents included:
  - standard operating procedures for recruitment, training and financial processes;
  - partnership agreement specifying roles and contributions;
  - tools to aid a scoping exercise and the collection of baseline data about PPIE activity;
  - consolidated set of key performance indicators;
  - a pilot instrument to help measure the impact of PPIE activity.

- Research partners were asked to produce first drafts of several of these documents. The group's membership was mainly from within the centre but included advisory membership from Health and Social Care Wales and Involve (invo.org.uk). The current chair of Involve acts as an external mentor and is a member of the PPIE group.

- A small annual budget was agreed to offer expenses and honoraria to the theme research partners at nationally recommended rates. Research partners were each given 'time budgets' of up to 10 half-days annually for which they might claim. Some of the research partners claim for their time; others do so only intermittently or not at all.

Successes

The early decisions referred to above were crucial to setting both the tone and strategic direction of the development of PPIE in the centre. Perhaps more than anything else the leadership and commitment offered at the most senior levels of the organization and the adoption of a supportive, problem solving approach to PPIE were key to any success achieved. Importantly, this approach was also exemplified on a daily basis by the behaviour of the research partners and research leads of the various projects, and the mutual appreciation of their respective contributions.

More practically, we produced a suite of documents and processes to cover all aspects of the implementation of PPIE in order to support researchers and research partners in their practice. These documents were intended to comprise generic content that could be adapted as needed for the diverse work of the themes. It was helpful to have a set of key performance indicators to help gauge progress over time. To stay on target, we used a strategic timeline of core events with a form of project management (PRINCE2 Lite) to register any piece of work we undertook, deadlines, dependencies, and a traffic light system so that we could see immediately anything at risk of non-completion. Our outline targets for the first 12 months of the project are shown in Figure 18.1. More recently, we have developed a separate Gantt chart to keep track of the work being undertaken within the themes by research partners and researchers. The research partners submit online diaries of activity and report to the PPIE group with subsequent collation of activities on an individual and collective basis.

The role that the research partners undertake in the centre is probably quite unlike that traditionally undertaken by members of the public in cancer research. While research partners do, on request, comment on protocols and other documents, their primary role, as already indicated, is strategic: to co-lead on the filling of gaps in, and dismantling obstacles to, further progress on PPIE. Examples of projects currently being undertaken are the development of tools to support members of the public fresh to their ambassadorial role in cancer research, developing a tool to measure the impact of PPIE, helping to recruit more patients to research and trying to expand the pool of research partners available to different themes. It is hoped that appraisals of these projects can be published and made available to researchers and research partners more widely.

This enhanced role of research partners has made it even more important than usual to recruit people with the right skills and backgrounds to the roles of theme research partners. The roles were advertised widely in Wales against role descriptions and appointment criteria, and candidates were appointed by panels of the researchers with whom they would be working, as well as by the lead research partner and researcher. Each theme research partner is asked to sign up to a partnership agreement which sets out the respective roles and expectations of researchers and research partners and the ways in which they would work together. The research partners have nominated mentors and the opportunity to discuss progress with them on a quarterly basis, although contact happens more frequently than that, in person, by phone or by email. Many of the theme research partners have contributed to the development of these ways of working by their membership of the PPIE group and are supportive of them.

It is important to stress that the research partners are working in fertile ground. The scoping exercise revealed large amounts of very good PPIE practice by clinicians and researchers, sometimes without identifying the work as PPIE, and has found them welcoming and willing partners in their roles.

Challenges

The main challenges in this project have been about time. The lay lead is an unpaid volunteer, committed to working for up to 1 day a week; in many weeks in the first 2 years, 1 day has stretched to 3. The lead academic has no protected time and has undertaken the role in her spare time. Most recently, she has formally adopted PPIE as one of her research themes and as part of her substantive role, funded by Marie Curie. In the first 12 months, both leads worked intensively, meeting at least weekly, to develop and refine implementation processes. The other key member of the lead PPIE team is a highly skilled administrator; she also commits more than the 1 day a week allocated and at a much higher level than an ordinary administrator. As already indicated, at least some of the theme research partners work well beyond the time allocated; they do this because they enjoy the role and can see the difference it makes. The biggest time deficit, however, resides with the researchers and clinicians in the Wales Cancer Research Centre. Very few, if any, have built into their job description any core allowance for PPIE activity. As one example of good practice,

Establish PPIE advisory group, April 2015	We wrote role descriptions for PPIE research partners We invited expressions of interest for PPIE theme research partners We appointed one lead research partner
Scoping current practice	We designed a scoping tool and assessed existing PPIE activity across all areas of the WCRC We met the theme and work package leads and assessed the feasibility of each area of further PPIE
Initiating	Our baseline scoping results were presented to the PPIE advisory group We interviewed and appointed two research partners per theme
Training	We used the existing MCPCRC/WCTU training model for our new research partners We asked a research partner to develop a generic PPIE SOP for both research partners and researchers
Performance monitoring	We asked a research partner to develop ways of measuring the impact of PPIE We will repeat annual scoping of PPIE activity within each theme and present the findings at the annual WCRC meetings
PPIE recruitment	We are working with other volunteers and NHS groups to develop a large pool of potential research partners
Governance	We hold weekly progress review meetings We work to tight budgets, with most members of the advisory group contributing time from their paid roles, or entirely voluntarily
Dissemination	We circulate a quarterly PPIE newsletter to the advisory group and external stakeholders We plan to publish our work as a protocol paper in 2017
Impact	We are piloting an impact measurement tool in a full study about the needs of bereaved carers A second study 'HIDDEN', which screens patients in the hospice for blood clots, is about to further test this tool

Figure 18.1 PPIE key activities during the first 12 months. MCPCRC, Marie Curie Palliative Care Research Centre; SOP, standard operating procedure; WCRC, Wales Cancer Research Centre; WCTU, Wales Cancer Trials Unit.

however, the Marie Curie Centre has adopted PPIE as custom and practice of any researcher/administration roles by specifying PPIE objectives in job descriptions for new appointments and as appraisal objectives for all team members.

Other research teams mostly do what they can out of goodwill. Until funders, be that government agencies or charities, recognize the centrality of PPIE to research by funding it, it will tend to remain an underfunded and fringe activity.

Conclusion

 There is much work to be done in establishing an effective and replicable PPIE framework, supported by an evidence base of evaluation and impact measurement. Further research to develop and test new initiatives is vital, the most important being research around 'impact'. Does PPIE make a difference? Where is it valuable? What does it change?

It is clear from the project that PPIE is both valuable and appreciated. There is anecdotal evidence of the impact it makes. Funders are less tolerant of 'lip service' attempts at PPIE and demand a far more considered approach. To be given full credibility, to be replicable, and to be taken seriously in the research community, however, PPIE as an intervention needs to be given the time for implementation and the tools for evaluation of its impact and effectiveness, as rigorously as any other research or clinical service development process.

CASE STUDY

01 A Young Adult with Sarcoma: a Case of Complexities

Anna Olsson-Brown, Jane Younger

Case history

A 23-year-old Polish woman presented as an emergency with back pain and was found to be in urinary retention. Investigations showed a large pelvic mass and innumerable lung metastases that were shown on biopsy to be a form of rhabdomyosarcoma. She was admitted for emergency chemotherapy to the regional teenage and young adult (TYA) unit. The intense chemotherapy regimen of ifosfamide, vincristine, dactinomycin and doxorubicin (IVADO), and vincristine, ifosfamide, doxorubicin and etoposide (VIDE) has a rapid induction and then runs over a 6 month period. The regimen is highly challenging, with immediate implementation and long periods of inpatient admission; it is very commonly associated with multiple complications such as neutropenic sepsis.

From the initial encounter there were significant barriers to communication, and a lability of engagement associated with fluctuation in mood, acceptance of therapy and interaction with the TYA cancer medicine team. There were additional challenges given the differences in cultural customs in the UK compared with Poland and while there was not an apparent language barrier in this case the difference in approach posed significant challenges for our patient.

As her treatment continued it emerged that there were numerous events occurring within her family and social setting that were affecting her acceptance and engagement with treatment. This led to variable compliance with significant medications and manifestation of a, likely premorbid, eating disorder which contributed to deterioration of her performance status. These events also significantly limited her ability to cope with her diagnosis and treatment, and the impact intense chemotherapy was having on her life and relationships.

She had ongoing input from an experienced TYA multidisciplinary team (MDT) throughout her treatment, which proved invaluable, and through provision of support from multiple avenues she was able to optimize her experience of treatment and work through the external issues that were having such a significant impact on her throughout treatment.

Background

Why are psychosocial issues commonly seen in TYA patients with cancer?

What steps can be taken to support TYA patients?

What is the role of the MDT?

How is depression in children and young people managed?

Background

Cancer in young people is rare. The incidence in the UK is 269 cases per million young people (aged 16–24 years), which accounted for 2214 new cases of cancer between 2008 and 2010.[1] The needs of young people are significant and diverse, and require specific input, therapy management structures and support mechanisms. This is particularly the case as they are, as a group, generally looked after within the adult healthcare sector. These requirements have been embedded within the NHS via the production and implementation of NICE guidance.[1,2]

Why are psychosocial issues commonly seen in TYA patients with cancer?

During their formative years teenagers and young people develop extensively not only physically but also emotionally, socially and psychologically. Even in the absence of a cancer diagnosis, it is a challenging time, when young people question the status quo and begin to develop their own values and beliefs. This can cause conflict with parents and family members, struggles with rules and boundaries, fluctuations in thought processes, and development of complex dynamics in friendships and relationships; it can often result in risk taking.[1,3]

When cancer treatment, be it curative or palliative, is added to the situation, careful and comprehensive support and management are essential. Regression is also commonly observed in

Table 1.1 Reciprocal effects of chronic illness and adolescent development.[3]

Effects of chronic illness on development	Effects of developmental issues on chronic illness or disability
Biological • Delayed puberty • Short stature • Reduced bone mass accretion	**Biological** • Increased calorific requirement for growth may negatively impact on disease parameters • Pubertal hormones may impact on disease parameters
Psychological • Infantilization • Adoption of the sick role as a personal identifier • Egocentricity persists into late adolescence • Impaired development of a sense of sexual or attractive self	**Poor adherence** • Poorly developed abstract thinking and planning • Reduced ability to plan and prepare • Difficulty in imagining the future; self-concept as being 'bullet-proof' • Rejection of medical professionals as part of separation from parents • Exploratory (risk-taking) behaviours
Social • Reduced independence at a time when independence is normally developing • Failure of peer relationships and intimate (couple) relationships • Social isolation • Educational failure and potential for vocational failure • Failure of development of independent living ability	**Associated health risk behaviours** • Chaotic eating habits may result in poor nutrition • Smoking, alcohol and drug use, often in excess of normal population rates • Sexual risk taking, possibly in view of realization of limited lifespan

TYA patients (Table 1.1). Furthermore, as a young person progresses through the care pathway it is likely that their needs and the needs of those around them will change.

What steps can be taken to support TYA patients?

A number of steps can be taken to support TYA patients during diagnosis and treatment of cancer.

- Young people and their families should have their care needs assessed and acted upon at key points in the care pathway, resulting in regular re-evaluation.
- There should be open communication and involvement of TYA patients in treatment discussions and decision-making processes.
- Recognize that their relationships with their parents and friends, and in some cases their children, will be complex and there will be multiple differences of opinion on many matters of care. This can lead to emotional challenges and conflict; therefore, developing proficient and sensitive conflict resolution skills is important.
- TYA patients should be supported to maintain as many of their normal activities as possible, including education if appropriate.
- Accept and understand that many of their responses to diagnosis or events during treatment are a normal way of coping and processing information at this stage of life.
- Develop an environment where young adults can talk to one another and form a degree of peer support.

NICE recommends psychological and social assessment of the following needs: age-appropriate patient information and coping skills; family information and coping skills; financial support; practical support; social and cultural circumstances; education and employment; the needs of siblings; relationships with peers; and spiritual needs.[1] Key assessment points in the cancer care pathway are: at diagnosis; during treatment; at the end of treatment; during long-term follow-up; at relapse; during palliative care; and following bereavement (for families and carers).[1]

What is the role of the MDT?

Effective treatment requires a combined approach to management focusing on medical and psychosocial aspects of care. The treatment of all young people with cancer should be discussed and coordinated by two MDTs including a cancer site-specific MDT and a TYA MDT. Two MDTs are needed in order to agree and deliver the appropriate treatment while ensuring that patients and families are supported physically, emotionally, psychologically and socially.

Core members of a TYA MDT include: lead clinician; consultants with clinical practice in cancer sites commonly affecting young people, including haematological malignancies, germ cell tumours and sarcomas, together with a clinical nurse specialist in malignancies; paediatric oncologist; principal treatment centre lead nurse; TYA clinical nurse specialist; psychologist or level 3 psychology support worker; young people's social worker; youth worker/activity coordinator; TYA key worker; MDT coordinator/secretary; others, such as palliative care team representative, physiotherapist, dietitian, TYA radiographer, and member of staff from the TYA unit.[1,4]

The TYA MDT is constructed to ensure that the young patient's needs can always be met and there is a team of individuals who know the patient's history and can be called upon when needed. This allows the patient to be effectively managed by a large number of people without finding it threatening or unpleasant. In the large part this leads to young people feeling supported, which can aid treatment significantly. Additionally, part of the purpose of the TYA MDT meeting is to discuss and propose interventions that are needed even when there is no requirement for a specific change in cancer treatment but there are issues that must be addressed concerning the patient's holistic needs and well-being.

Psychological support

Psychological support can be provided by all members of the team. The degree of support provided is classically divided into levels (Table 1.2).[5] A trained clinical psychologist's level of input is variable and is based on the requirements of each individual patient. Not all patients cared for by the TYA MDT will require the support of a clinical psychologist and their input is flexible over time. Within the team, clinical psychologists have a number of roles including assessment of needs, home visits, patient and family support and development of a psychologist/key worker interface. In doing so they are able to provide support and non-pharmacological management strategies to promote the psychological well-being of TYA patients.

Charities

CLIC Sargent (www.clicsargent.org.uk) is a cancer charity for children and young people. It provides support for teenagers and young people with cancer at a national level in a number of areas. The main areas of focus include: reducing the practical and financial impact of cancer treatment; supporting emotional well-being and resilience; supporting family life and maximizing time spent safely at home during treatment; and enabling access to education, training and employment.

The Teenage Cancer Trust (www.teenagecancertrust.org) is dedicated to providing specialist care and support to young people with cancer. It provides TYA specialist facilities in hospitals across the UK; funds specialist nurses and youth support coordinators; provides outreach support enabling young patients to receive optimal access to support irrespective of where they live; supports activities for young people with cancer to promote social support and growth; provides real-hair wigs for every young person with cancer; and provides education to young people in order to promote early detection of cancer.

How is depression in young people managed?

The use of antidepressants in the TYA population should be considered especially carefully.

Children and young adults aged ≤18 years

No antidepressants are licensed for use in children (≤18 years of age). NICE guidelines for depression in children and young people recommend psychological intervention for mild depression.[6] Patients with moderate or severe depression should be referred to child and adolescent mental health services. NICE recommends that these patients should be offered a specific psychological intervention before considering using antidepressant medication combined with psychological treatment. It is important in the under-18 population that the risk of suicide is assessed and that suicidal ideas are monitored when treating for depression. NICE guidelines

Table 1.2 Healthcare professionals who provide different levels of psychological support.[5]

Level of support	Professional provider
1	Any healthcare professional
2	A clinical nurse specialist trained to provide a holistic needs assessment
3	Trained councillor
4	Clinical psychologist/psychiatrist

recommend fluoxetine as the antidepressant of choice; second line treatment includes sertraline and citalopram.[6]

Young adults aged 19–24

In the over-18 population, NICE recommends that for mild or sub-threshold depression psychological therapies are offered in the first instance, but for those who do not respond and for moderate depression antidepressants may be offered.[6] It is thought that in the under-25 population, there is an increased risk of suicide with antidepressant treatment, similar to that seen in under 18s.[7] It is therefore important to assess suicide risk before prescribing, and then continue to monitor this risk while the patient remains on medication.

Conclusion and learning points

- The management of TYA patients with cancer is complex and multifaceted.
- The normal physiological and emotional changes which occur during a person's formative years add to the challenges faced by TYA cancer patients.
- There is an established framework of assessment to ensure that the needs of TYA cancer patients (and their families) are being met.
- Young patients with cancer are supported by a large MDT, each member of which has a specific and unique focus to optimize patient care.
- Depression is a common condition affecting TYA cancer patients. NICE guidance recommends the implementation of psychological intervention prior to pharmacological intervention in this group.

References

1 National Institute for Health and Care Excellence (2014). *Cancer services for children and young people. Quality standard QS55.* Available from: www.nice.org.uk/guidance/qs55 (accessed 14 July 2017).

2 National Institute for Health and Care Excellence. *Improving outcomes in children and young people with cancer.* London: NICE, 2005.

3 Michaud P-A, Suris JC, Viner R. *The adolescent with a chronic condition: epidemiology, developmental issues and health care provision.* Geneva: WHO, 2007.

4 Smith S, Case L, Waterhouse K, *et al. A blueprint of care for teenagers and young adults with cancer.* Manchester: Teenage Cancer Trust, 2014.

5 National Institute for Health and Care Excellence. *Improving supportive and palliative care for adults with cancer.* London: NICE, 2004.

6 National Institute for Health and Care Excellence. *Depression in children and young people: identification and management. Clinical guideline CG28.* London: NICE, 2005 (updated 2015).

7 McGorry P, Birleson P. Should youth mental health become a speciality in its own right? *BMJ* 2009; 339: 834–5.

02 Cancer of Unknown Primary Treated with Palliative Chemotherapy and Hospice Care

Nicola Hughes, Daniel Swinson, Emma Lowe

Case history

A 70-year-old man, with a medical history of hypertension only, presented to his GP with a 2 month history of cough, early satiety, abdominal bloating and reduced appetite. A chest X-ray showed bilateral pleural effusions. A subsequent CT scan demonstrated widespread omental and peritoneal disease. Bilateral pulmonary emboli were also present.

He was reviewed in the cancer of unknown primary clinic, where he was commenced on low-molecular-weight heparin and referred for omental biopsy and ascitic drainage. Histopathology and immunohistochemistry confirmed a mucinous adenocarcinoma with positive expression of cytokeratin (CK) 7, patchy expression of homeobox protein CDX2, and negative expression of CK-20, prostate-specific antigen and thyroid transcription factor 1 (TTF-1). Abnormal tumour markers included CA-19.9 of 16,473 and carcinoembryonic antigen (CEA) 11.

An endoscopy found a tumour in the second part of the duodenum (D2), consistent with a primary small bowel cancer. After discussion at the multidisciplinary team (MDT) meeting and review in the gastrointestinal oncology clinic, treatment with oxaliplatin, fluorouracil and folinic acid (OxMdG) chemotherapy with an intermittent approach (treat for a fixed period with planned re-challenge on progression) was offered. The patient completed two programmes of OxMdG; however, during the third he began to deteriorate. He was deemed unsuitable for second line chemotherapy and was referred for the Gold Standards Framework (goldstandardsframework.org.uk).

The following month he had two admissions with vomiting and aspiration pneumonia. Discussions with the patient in the presence of his wife and son disclosed that his prognosis was in the order of a short number of weeks. He was reviewed by the palliative care team, who documented that he was aware that he was approaching the end of his life. He expressed a strong wish for end-of-life intravenous fluid support and his preferred place of death was the local hospice. He was transferred to the hospice the following week. Soon after arriving, however, he became unhappy with the care he was receiving. He requested administration of intravenous fluids, which resulted in pulmonary oedema and ascites. The patient was not able to recall he had been told that he was approaching the end of his life. The hospice team contacted the oncology team, requesting that he be transferred back to the hospital according to his wishes. Discussions took place between the treating teams and he returned to the hospital.

On his return to hospital he stated that he wanted to be 'actively managed', including total parenteral nutrition, as he felt he was being starved. He was able to tolerate oral fluids, and, after long discussions with him, intravenous fluids were limited to 1 l/day. He sadly died 10 days after returning from the hospice.

What are the positive and negative factors associated with intravenous fluids at the end of life?

What are the ethical and legal issues surrounding the use of intravenous fluids at the end of life?

When should intravenous fluids be used at the end of life?

What is the role of subcutaneous fluids at the end of life?

Was he prescribed the most appropriate chemotherapy?

What are the positive and negative factors associated with intravenous fluids at the end of life?

One of the challenges of prescribing intravenous fluids at the end of life is the lack of any evidence of benefit. A randomized controlled trial by Bruera et al.[1] found no statistically significant difference in overall survival in hospice patients receiving 1 l/day compared with 100 ml/day 0.9% saline intravenous fluid. No difference was found between groups in the incidence of delirium or symptoms of dehydration (fatigue, myoclonus, sedation and hallucinations). An improvement in symptoms was reported by both patient groups on day 4, suggesting a possible placebo effect. The lack of overall efficacy is supported by a recently updated Cochrane review.[2]

Other negative factors include the need to maintain intravenous access and potential need for a catheter, both of which may cause the patient additional discomfort. The risk of electrolyte disturbance may increase the use of blood tests at the end of life. The patient is also at an increased risk of oedema, ascites and pleural effusions, and the potentially unpleasant symptoms associated with these comorbidities. A Japanese study, however, found that fluid retention did not impact on a patient's quality of life in this setting.[3]

Maintaining hydration may be perceived by patients and relatives as a means to enhance comfort and dignity. In this respect it provides a symptomatic benefit, even if it is a placebo effect. There may also be a perception that intravenous fluids will stop the patient feeling thirsty. Thirst in patients at the end of life has been found to be multifactorial and associated with overall poor health, stomatitis, oral breathing and use of opiates.[4] Artificial hydration may therefore not alleviate the symptom and adequate mouth care may be more effective.

There is undoubtedly a role for administration of intravenous fluids in patients with dysphagia or complete bowel obstruction. By providing hydration, artificially unpleasant symptoms, such as vomiting, are prevented by avoiding attempts at oral intake. Additional hydration may also help prevent or limit the build-up of metabolites and medications.

What are the ethical and legal issues surrounding the use of intravenous fluids at the end of life?

The provision of intravenous fluids at the end of life provides the treating medical team with an ethical dilemma, particularly in cases such as that presented here. The General Medical Council guidance states: 'Nutrition and hydration provided by a tube or a drip are regarded in law as medical treatment and should be treated in the same way as other medical interventions.'[5] In this respect the provision of fluids is ultimately a medical decision and if clinically indicated should be prescribed. We are duty-bound to practise within the ethical framework of beneficence and non-maleficence. Fluids, however, are often regarded as a basic need that should not be withdrawn. When a patient requests intravenous fluids, and has the capacity to do so, we must therefore accept the patient's autonomy and beliefs.

When should intravenous fluids be used at the end of life?

When deciding whether or not a patient should receive intravenous fluids at the end of life, the treating team needs to consider the risks and benefits in respect of each individual patient. The patient's own wishes and the wishes of the family, especially if the patient lacks capacity, need to be taken into account, along with any predefined care goals. If there is disagreement between the patient's and/or family's wishes and that of the medical team then a full discussion of the potential risks needs to take place and should be clearly documented. It may also be beneficial to explore why the patient wants fluids to be provided and to address any false beliefs. It is important to reassure the patient and those close to them that he or she will continue to receive a high quality of care, particularly with regards to any distressing symptoms that may develop, even if fluids are not provided.

What is the role of subcutaneous fluids at the end of life?

Subcutaneous fluids are often underused at the end of life, due to reliance on the intravenous route, but they can provide a useful alternative. Subcutaneous fluids have been shown to be as effective as intravenous fluids in mild-to-moderate dehydration[6] and are associated with fewer complications, mainly due to no intravenous access being required. As not all hospices are able to give intravenous fluids, the use of the subcutaneous route may allow a patient to have end-of-life care in a hospice rather than a hospital.

Was he prescribed the most appropriate chemotherapy?

This patient was treated with systemic chemotherapy for metastatic duodenal cancer, after MDT discussion deemed this was the most likely origin of his cancer. Cancers of the small intestine are rare and account for around 2–3% of gastrointestinal tumours. Prognosis is poor and, due to the non-specific nature of its presentation, patients, as in this case, often present at an advanced stage.

Owing to a lack of randomized data, no standard chemotherapy regimen currently exists for the treatment of metastatic small bowel cancer. Treatment is therefore largely extrapolated from the management of cancers of the large intestine. Existing evidence is limited to small phase II clinical trials or retrospective studies. A small phase II study of oxaliplatin and capecitabine reported a response rate of 50% and median survival of 20.4 months.[7] The efficacy of this regimen has been confirmed by single institutions and multicentre studies.

An international study evaluating the use of OxMdG in the adjuvant setting for small bowel adenocarcinoma is ongoing (Phase III Trial Investigating the Potential Benefit of Adjuvant Chemotherapy for Small Bowel Adenocarcinoma [BALLAD]) and may provide a stronger evidence base for the use of this regimen in this cancer type, accepting that this is for patients with earlier stage disease.

Conclusion and learning points

- A patient-centred approach should be taken to intravenous fluid administration at the end of life.

- Subcutaneous fluids provide a useful alternative route for artificial hydration at the end of life.

References

1 Bruera E, Hui D, Dalal S, *et al*. Parenteral hydration in patients with advanced cancer: a multicentre, double-blind, placebo-controlled randomized trial. *J Clin Oncol* 2013; 31: 111–18.

2 Good P, Richard R, Syrmis W, *et al*. Medically assisted hydration for adult palliative care patients. *Cochrane Database Syst Rev* 2014; 4: CD006273.

3 Yamaguchi T, Morita T, Shinjo T, *et al*. Effect of parenteral hydration therapy based on the Japanese national clinical guideline on quality of life, discomfort and symptom intensity in patients with advanced cancer. *J Pain Symptom Manage* 2012; 43: 1001–12.

4 Morita T, Tei Y, Tsunoda J, *et al*. Determinants of the sensation of thirst in terminally ill cancer patients. *Support Care Cancer* 2001; 9: 177.

5 General Medical Council (2010). *End of life care: clinically assisted nutrition and hydration*. Available from: www.gmc-uk.org/guidance/ethical_guidance/end_of_life_clinically_assisted_nutrition_and_hydration.asp (accessed 5 March 2017).

6 Arinzon Z, Feldman J, Fidelman Z, *et al*. Hypodermoclysis (subcutaneous infusion) effective mode of treatment of dehydration in long-term care patients. *Arch Gerontol Geriatr* 2004; 38: 167–73.

7 Overman MJ, Varadhachary GR, Kopetz S, *et al*. Phase II study of capecitabine and oxaliplatin for advanced adenocarcinoma of the small bowel and ampulla of Vater. *J Clin Oncol* 2009; 27: 2598–603.

Further reading

- Zaanan A. Chemotherapy of advanced small bowel adenocarcinoma: a multicentre AGEO study. *Ann Oncol* 2010; 21: 1786–93.

03 A Patient with Advanced Oesophageal Cancer Requiring Interventional Radiology and Palliative Care Input

Mark Openshaw, Sam Khan, Meera Chauhan, Laura Clipsham, Anne Thomas

Case history

A 76-year-old man presented to a follow-up oncology clinic with symptoms of weight loss and severe reflux. He had previously received neoadjuvant epirubicin, cisplatin and capecitabine, and a subtotal gastrectomy for a T3N1M0 (4/4 lymph nodes) adenocarcinoma of the lower oesophagus. Asymptomatic mediastinal lymph node relapse occurred 3 years previously. He was currently under surveillance having received no palliative chemotherapy or radiotherapy. A CT scan following this appointment showed no progression of disease, and he was referred to palliative care for symptom control.

Symptoms of reflux had developed following surgery and were associated with anorexia. Although present during the day, they were worse at night. Anxiety regarding symptoms and the impact on quality of life (QOL) resulted in the patient stating he did not see the point of carrying on. At his palliative care appointment, the following medication changes were made:

- Continue esomeprazole 20 mg OD.
- Increase ranitidine to 150 mg BD.
- Start mebeverine 150 mg TDS.
- Start mirtazapine 7.5 mg ON.

A discussion with the gastroenterology team was undertaken regarding his symptoms. Gastric outlet obstruction was queried, resulting in the following changes in medication:

- Stop mebeverine.
- Start domperidone 10 mg TDS.

His imaging and history were reviewed at the gastroenterology multidisciplinary team meeting, at which mild gastric outlet obstruction secondary to coeliac axis lymphadenopathy was diagnosed. He was suitable for radiotherapy and received 20 Gy in five fractions of radiotherapy to that area.

Reflux persisted for 1 month after radiotherapy but improved when esomeprazole was increased to 40 mg/day.

Three months later he presented to his GP with persistent vomiting, breathlessness and weight loss. His GP requested a chest X-ray (Figure 3.1), which was initially

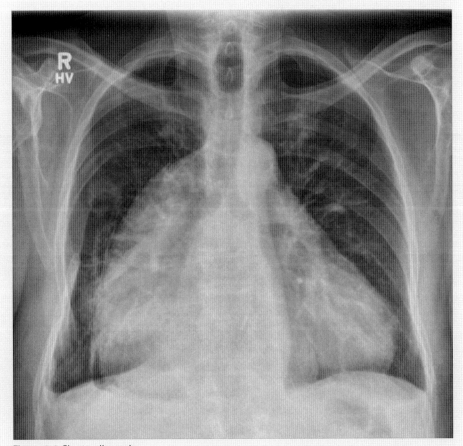

Figure 3.1 Chest radiograph.

interpreted as cardiomegaly, through failure to consider his surgical history. At his
oncology appointment a CT scan was requested, which demonstrated gastric outlet
obstruction with significant distension of the gastric conduit (Figure 3.2). His case
was discussed at the weekly radiology meeting and deemed suitable for stenting of
the obstruction. The risks and benefits of immediate nasogastric tube placement
versus planned stenting were discussed. The patient opted for planned inpatient
stenting. He was discharged after a 3 day stay and stent insertion. Three months
later he was well and required no further intervention.

What was the goal of cancer treatment for this patient? What is the evidence
base for further chemotherapeutic interventions for this patient?

Why is it important to take medical/surgical history into account when
requesting imaging?

What is the evidence for the change of treatment enacted by palliative care
and why was it changed following a potential diagnosis of gastric outlet
obstruction?

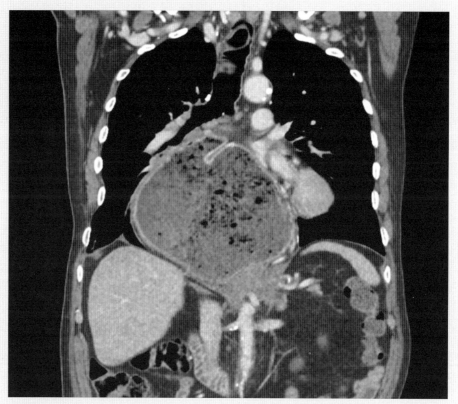

Figure 3.2 CT scan showing gastric outlet obstruction caused by malignant disease involving the lymph nodes.

What were the risks of delayed nasogastric tube placement? And when is radiotherapy preferred over stent placement for gastric outlet obstruction?

How can admissions for cancer patients in the last year of life be reduced?

What was the goal of cancer treatment for this patient? What is the evidence base for further chemotherapeutic interventions for this patient?

The goal of cancer treatment for this patient was primarily improvement of QOL and symptom control, with the secondary aim of extending life.

There is ongoing debate as to whether palliative chemotherapy extends life in patients with metastatic oesophageal cancer.[1] As a result, treatment focuses on patient symptoms, and chemotherapy is reserved for patients in whom symptoms are the result of disease progression that cannot be controlled by non-chemotherapeutic measures.

There is no standard second line therapy for patients with oesophageal cancer. For selected patients who have relapsed following combination therapy, a re-challenge with platinum plus fluoropyrimidine, with or without epirubicin, is indicated.[2] This is most beneficial for patients whose treatment was at least 12 months previously.

The Symptom Control with or without Docetaxel in Treating Patients with Relapsed

Oesophageal Cancer or Stomach Cancer (COUGAR-02) study showed that treatment with docetaxel improves median overall survival by approximately 2 months,[3] and it is therefore frequently used as a second line chemotherapy agent. Global health-related quality-of-life measures were similar whether treatment was or was not received, but disease-specific measurements such as abdominal pain and dysphagia were improved.

The patient in question therefore had further chemotherapeutic options; however, because he presented with symptoms specific to the primary recurrent tumour, direct therapy to the tumour such as radiotherapy and tumour stenting were indicated in preference to chemotherapy.

Why is it important to take medical/surgical history into account when requesting imaging?

This case presents a strong message regarding the importance of relevant history when requesting investigations. The chest radiograph in Figure 3.1 may at first glance be consistent with cardiomegaly due to cardiac failure, but on closer inspection the right heart border is clearly visible showing that this is not the case. This patient had had a subtotal gastrectomy with gastric pull-through. In light of this important part of the history, it is apparent that the appearance of the chest radiograph is due to enlargement of the gastric conduit. Had this information been available to the reporting radiologist, there would have been a far lower chance of an initial misreporting of the abnormality and timelier referral to oncology. This case therefore highlights the importance of putting relevant surgical history on image requests, and of ensuring GPs are aware of important oncological history by providing relevant information in patient letters.

What is the evidence for the change of treatment enacted by palliative care and why was it changed following a potential diagnosis of gastric outlet obstruction?

Discomfort and distress due to the symptoms of reflux are common in patients with oesophageal cancer. Esomeprazole is a proton pump inhibitor that reduces acid secretion and is widely used to treat reflux. Ranitidine is a histamine H2-antagonist that has an anti-secretory effect and reduces acid production. Both of these actions help reduce symptoms of reflux and act synergistically with a proton pump inhibitor. The optimal dose for ranitidine is 150 mg BD, which therefore required dose escalation. Mebeverine is a smooth muscle relaxant which, by relaxing the muscles of the stomach and lower oesophagus, can reduce reflux symptoms.

Following a potential diagnosis of a partial gastric outlet obstruction, muscle relaxants should be avoided, as they will reduce the ability of the gastrointestinal tract to push the intestinal contents past the narrowing. A prokinetic such as domperidone is instead indicated. When adjusting medications, one should first optimize the medication that a patient is taking, ensuring the correct dose and most efficient route of administration. Combining medications for synergistic effect can then be enacted if symptoms are inadequately controlled. The palliative care team is best placed to provide advice on management of complex symptoms.

What were the risks of delayed nasogastric tube placement? And when is radiotherapy preferred over stent placement for gastric outlet obstruction?

The patient was informed of the risks of delaying stomach aspiration, the main risk being that of regurgitation of stomach contents and subsequent aspiration. Of note, although nasogastric tube placement reduces the chance of food aspiration it does not abolish the risk of aspiration of secretions. By keeping the patient informed he remained at the centre of decision making and he elected to avoid emergency admission.

The management of malignant gastric outlet obstruction is both limited and controversial. Surgical treatment of gastric outlet obstruction is via a gastrojejunostomy. Studies have shown that although surgical intervention can result in higher levels of nausea and a longer hospital stay in comparison with endoscopic intervention, there is considerable improvement in long-term symptomatic relief, with low rates of re-intervention.[4] As the benefit is long term but the increased risks are short term, surgical intervention is recommended only for those with a longer life expectancy.

There are few studies that directly compare the benefits of a stent versus a gastrojejunostomy. Studies highlight the high rate of short-term symptomatic relief, the minimally invasive technique and the improvement in QOL associated with a stent insertion, and recommend consideration of a stent placement in those with a life expectancy of less than 2–6 months.[5]

External beam radiotherapy is a minimally invasive technique that can also be used to treat gastric outlet obstruction. Radiotherapy has the advantage of relieving symptoms and also reducing tumour burden. The response to radiotherapy is not as immediate as with more invasive techniques, but studies in gastric cancer show that at 1 month follow-up, over 50% of patients treated still had relief of obstructive symptoms, and the treatment was well tolerated.[6] There are currently no studies that directly compare radiotherapy with stent placement or surgery.

How can admissions for cancer patients in the last year of life be reduced?

Members of the public, when asked about good end-of-life care, have previously identified person-centred care as important, including supporting patient choice.[7] Shared decision making is an important part of advance care planning for patients who may be in the last year of life, and is supported by open, honest discussions about the patient's phase of illness and anticipated deterioration. Advance care planning explores patients' priorities and wishes for their care and can avoid unwanted or unnecessary hospital admissions. It usually takes place in anticipation of a deterioration in the patient's condition in the future, either in loss of capacity or in ability to communicate wishes to others.[8] By identifying patients with cancer who may be in the last year of life, initiating these discussions and documenting them, admissions may be reduced by supporting patients to get 'the right care, at the right time, in the right setting, from the right caregivers'.[9] Use of the 'surprise question' ('Would you be surprised if this patient were to die in the next few weeks, months or days?') can help actively identify patients nearing the end of their life and trigger specific and proactive support to ensure they 'live well until they die'.[10]

Conclusion and learning points

- Palliative chemotherapy for patients with oesophageal cancer is available but its use should be balanced with the risks and benefits of other available disease and symptom control methods, with the primary aim of improving QOL.

- Providing relevant medical and surgical history is essential for correctly interpreting diagnostic imaging.

- Understanding the mechanism of action of medication is important for controlling symptoms of reflux and gastric outlet obstruction. Optimizing these medications involves optimizing the dose and route of administration before combining medications.

- Nasogastric tube placement does not abolish the risk of aspiration from secretions.

- Stenting for gastric outlet obstruction is preferred over surgery, for patients with short life expectancy. Radiotherapy is preferred if immediate relief of symptoms is not required.

- Providing patient-centred care in the last year of life can be improved by identifying such patients and starting discussions on advance care planning. This can avoid unwanted or unnecessary hospital admissions.

- Use of the 'surprise question' can help identify patients in the last year of life.

References

1 Adenis A, Penel N, Horn S, *et al.* Palliative chemotherapy does not improve survival in metastatic esophageal cancer. *Oncology* 2010; 79: 46–54.

2 Okines AF, Asghar U, Cunningham D, *et al.* Rechallenge with platinum plus fluoropyrimidine +/− epirubicin in patients with oesophagogastric cancer. *Oncology* 2010; 79: 150–8.

3 Ford HER, Marshall A, Bridgewater JA, *et al.* Docetaxel versus active symptom control for refractory oesophagogastric adenocarcinoma (COUGAR-02): an open-label, phase 3 randomised controlled trial. *Lancet Oncol* 2014; 15: 78–86.

4 Jeurnink SM, Steyerberg EW, van Hooft JE, *et al.* Surgical gastrojejunostomy or endoscopic stent placement for the palliation of malignant gastric outlet obstruction (SUSTENT study): a multicenter randomized trial. *Gastrointest Endosc* 2010; 71: 490–9.

5 van Heek NT, van Geenen RC, Busch OR, Gouma DJ. Palliative treatment in 'peri'-pancreatic carcinoma: stenting or surgical therapy? *Acta Gastroenterol Belg* 2002; 65: 171–5.

6 Tey J, Choo BA, Leong CN, *et al.* Clinical outcome of palliative radiotherapy for locally advanced symptomatic gastric cancer in the modern era. *Medicine* 2014; 93: e118.

7 British Medical Association (2017). *End-of-life care and physician-assisted dying.* Available from: www.bma.org.uk/collective-voice/policy-and-research/ethics/end-of-life-care (accessed 28 February 2017).

8 NHS England (2008). *End of life care. Advance care planning: a guide for health and social care staff.* Available from: www.ncpc.org.uk/sites/default/files/AdvanceCarePlanning.pdf (accessed 20 February 2017).

9 The National Council for Palliative Care (2015). *Getting serious about prevention: enabling people to stay out of hospital at the end of life.* Available from: www.ncpc.org.uk/sites/default/files/Getting%20Serious_WEB.pdf (accessed 28 February 2017).

10 Royal College of General Practitioners (2011). *The GSF Prognostic Indicator Guidance.* Available from: www.goldstandardsframework.org.uk/cd-content/uploads/files/ General%20Files/Prognostic%20Indicator%20Guidance%20October%202011.pdf (accessed 28 February 2017).

04 A Metastatic Breast Cancer Patient Who Was Suicidal and Refused Treatment

Kok Haw Jonathan Lim, Bethan Daniel, Tracey Coleby, Andrew M. Wardley

Case history

A 53-year-old woman with metastatic breast cancer presented to hospital with worsening back pain and suicidal ideation. She had recently contacted the breast care nurses and her GP several times with non-cardiac chest pain, severe anxiety attacks and other non-specific symptoms. She had no other medical illnesses apart from depression, for which citalopram and diazepam had been prescribed. She was still working as a chief flight attendant. She was divorced and lived alone, but had a good relationship with her mother and a few close friends.

The patient was initially diagnosed with oestrogen receptor (ER)-positive human epidermal growth factor receptor 2 (HER2)-negative left breast carcinoma at age 38 years. Although radically treated, she subsequently relapsed with multifocal ipsilateral breast carcinoma 12 years later. Unfortunately, 2 years after her second adjuvant treatment, she developed metastatic liver and bone disease. She then progressed through four lines of treatment in short succession: tamoxifen; fulvestrant and a protein kinase B (Akt) inhibitor (Fulvestrant Akt Inhibition in Advanced Aromatase Inhibitor-Resistant Breast Cancer [FAKTION] trial); capecitabine; and everolimus and exemestane. She was devastated to learn about her most recent progression and did not turn up to any clinic appointments or engage with any members of her oncology team. She wanted to run away from facing her advanced, progressing disease. She feared further chemotherapy would disfigure her and make her look ill, and she would therefore lose her professional identity. This was compounded by her recent relationship breakdown and the news that her best friend had died of breast cancer. She also started having flashbacks of her two maternal aunts dying painfully from breast cancer in their forties. She felt overwhelmed. Indeed, she had formed plans on how she would commit suicide and considered Dignitas, but had been held back by the thought of hurting her loved ones.

During this acute admission, she was hypercalcaemic and had worsening liver function. She was managed medically and was urgently seen by the psycho-oncology team. She had a prolonged hospital stay and, after much consideration, decided to proceed with paclitaxel, with major input and support from the breast and palliative care nurses. At last follow-up, she had an excellent partial response to treatment and began coming to terms with her diagnosis.

What is the evidence behind recommending second and subsequent lines of chemotherapy in metastatic breast cancer?

What can you do if a patient decides not to have any further treatment?

Is there any practical guidance in managing patients with advanced, progressing disease?

Is there evidence for earlier supportive and palliative care in metastatic breast cancer?

How common is suicidal ideation and thoughts of euthanasia among patients with metastatic cancer?

What is the legal position regarding euthanasia in cancer patients in the UK?

What is the evidence behind recommending second and subsequent lines of chemotherapy in metastatic breast cancer?

Despite the remarkable progress seen in breast cancer treatments over the past 30 years, treatment beyond first line palliative chemotherapy, particularly in HER2-negative metastatic breast cancer, remains an issue of contention. Retrospective studies have previously demonstrated the benefit of successive lines of treatment following progression to first line chemotherapy, albeit with decreasing levels of response and clinical benefit rates.[1-3] In a recent prospective Korean study of 240 women with HER2-negative metastatic breast cancer, the median overall survival was 31.2 months and the median progression-free survival for first line, second line and third line chemotherapy was 7.6, 5.1 and 3.6 months, respectively.[4] Together with others,[2,5] Park *et al.*[4] have observed a correlation between response to previous chemotherapy and response to subsequent lines of treatment, especially if there has been a progression-free interval of more than 6–8 months following first line chemotherapy.

Above all, we know that patient selection remains pivotal and this is still generally assessed by performance status. The decision for more treatment should be made in partnership with the patient knowing that the main aim of treatment is to optimize quality of life (QOL) and in a few cases prolong overall survival.

What can you do if a patient decides not to have any further treatment?

In the UK, as set out in the good medical practice guidance issued by the General Medical Council, treatment decisions should be made in partnership between the doctor and the patient.[6] If the patient is deemed to have capacity, the patient's wishes should be respected even if they seem wrong or irrational to the doctor. It is the doctor's duty to provide adequate facts regarding the patient's condition, investigations required and treatment options, including having a balanced benefits-versus-risks discussion, in order to support the patient in making an informed decision.

For a patient who refuses treatment, the following applies:[6]

- Having a mental illness does not automatically call a patient's capacity into question and does not preclude the right to refuse treatment: Re C (Adult, refusal of treatment) [1994] 1 All ER 819.
- Capacity to refuse treatment must be time- and decision-specific: Re MB (Adult, medical treatment) [1997] 38 BMLR 175 CA.

• Right of a patient who has capacity to refuse life-prolonging treatment: Re B (Adult, refusal of medical treatment) [2002] 2 All ER 449.

Is there any practical guidance in managing patients with advanced, progressing disease?

There have been increasing efforts in recent years to address the evolving needs of patients with advanced, progressing cancer through national drives such as the National Confidential Enquiry into Patient Outcome and Death, end-of-life care strategy, the Gold Standards Framework, and preferred priorities for care. The management of these patients must be multidisciplinary to encompass their holistic needs in addition to their cancer. Here, the clinical nurse specialist is an essential key worker for the patient, providing continuity of care and coordinating input from the healthcare professionals involved. It is also recommended that advance care planning is discussed with the patient through closer communication between the hospital and community teams.

Is there evidence for earlier supportive and palliative care in metastatic breast cancer?

Randomized controlled trial data from both metastatic non-small-cell lung and gastrointestinal cancers indicate that early integration of palliative care improves QOL and the prevalence of depression and enables patients to be more open about their wishes.[7,8] More remarkably, earlier supportive and palliative care has been shown to independently improve survival in patients.[8,9] Moreover, it can help optimize the use of chemotherapy in advanced cancer by reducing the need for aggressive interventions in the last days or weeks of life.[10]

This promising observation can be translated into the care of patients with metastatic breast cancer. At The Christie NHS Foundation Trust we piloted the enhanced supportive care initiative to integrate earlier supportive and palliative care into the cancer care pathway, and it is now nationally funded by NHS England. Our preliminary audit results have shown a marked improvement in advanced cancer patients' opportunity to discuss their prognosis, and an objective reduction in the length of inpatient stays and fewer intensive care hospital days. This is projected not only to lower overall healthcare costs but also to improve patient outcomes.

How common is suicidal ideation and thoughts of euthanasia among patients with metastatic cancer?

It is difficult to obtain accurate objective data on such issues, as studies investigating suicide and euthanasia are undoubtedly both technically and ethically challenging, particularly in patients with metastatic cancer who are terminally ill. In a prospective cohort study in the Netherlands, where physician-assisted suicide is legal, van der Lee et al.[11] reported that at least 23% of their 138 cancer patients (estimated life expectancy of 3 months or less) had depressed mood and 22% had requested euthanasia (unprompted). They observed that those with depressed mood were four times more likely to express a wish for euthanasia.[11] This high prevalence of requests for euthanasia was also corroborated in another, more recent prospective study performed in the primary care setting in the Netherlands. Among 64 cancer patients with an estimated prognosis of 6 months or less, 27% had requested euthanasia and a third had proceeded with it.[12] Nevertheless, the prevalence of requests for euthanasia may be lower in countries where euthanasia is illegal. For example, in a large single-centre observational study of over 700 cancer patients receiving palliative care in Spain, only 2.5% had expressed thoughts of euthanasia.[13]

While 'unbearable suffering' remains the core justification for euthanasia, it is interesting to note that there is often no difference in the prevalence of suffering between those who request euthanasia and those who do not.[12,14] The decision to request euthanasia is always multifaceted and complex, but generally heavily influenced by socioeconomic factors, psychological state and religious belief.[14]

What is the legal position regarding euthanasia in cancer patients in the UK?

Under English law, regardless of any medical diagnosis or personal circumstances, all forms of euthanasia are illegal and are therefore not practised in the UK. Euthanasia may be considered manslaughter or murder and carry a sentence of life imprisonment. Although the act of suicide has been decriminalized, assisted suicide is punishable by the Suicide Act 1961 and carries a maximum penalty of up to 14 years' imprisonment.

Conclusion and learning points

- In well-selected patients with metastatic breast cancer, second and subsequent lines of palliative chemotherapy may be recommended with the aim of maintaining the patient's QOL.

- Any patient with capacity has the right to refuse treatment irrespective of any diagnosis of mental illness, and/or even if refusal of treatment results in death.

- The concept of enhanced supportive care is promising and has the potential to improve patients' QOL and survival outcomes.

- A considerably high percentage of metastatic cancer patients report depressed mood and express a wish for euthanasia, particularly in countries where euthanasia is legal.

- Any form of euthanasia or assisted suicide is illegal in the UK and punishable by law.

References

1 Tacca O, LeHeurteur M, Durando X, *et al.* Metastatic breast cancer: overall survival related to successive chemotherapies. What do we gain after the third line? *Cancer Invest* 2009; 27: 81–5.

2 Bonotto M, Gerratana L, Iacono D, *et al.* Treatment of metastatic breast cancer in a real-world scenario. Is progression-free survival with first line predictive of benefit from second and later lines? *Oncologist* 2015; 20: 719–24.

3 Bakker JL, Wever K, van Waesberghe JH, *et al.* What is the benefit of treatment with multiple lines of chemotherapy for patients with metastatic breast cancer? A retrospective cohort study. *Cancer Epidemiol* 2015; 39: 848–53.

4 Park IH, Lee KS, Ro J. Effects of second and subsequent lines of chemotherapy for metastatic breast cancer. *Clin Breast Cancer* 2015; 15: e55–62.

5 Banerji U, Kuciejewska A, Ashley S, *et al.* Factors determining outcome after third line chemotherapy for metastatic breast cancer. *Breast* 2007; 16: 359–66.

6 General Medical Council (2008). *Consent: patients and doctors making decisions together.* Available from: www.gmc-uk.org/Consent___English_1015.pdf_48903482.pdf (accessed 13 March 2017).

7 Temel JS, Greer JA, El-Jawahri A, *et al.* Effects of early integrated palliative care in patients with lung and GI cancer: a randomized clinical trial. *J Clin Oncol* 2017; 35: 834–41.

8 Temel JS, Greer JA, Muzikansky A, *et al.* Early palliative care for patients with metastatic non-small-cell lung cancer. *N Engl J Med* 2010; 363: 733–42.

9 Bakitas MA, Tosteson TD, Li Z, *et al.* Early versus delayed initiation of concurrent palliative oncology care: patient outcomes in the ENABLE III randomized controlled trial. *J Clin Oncol* 2015; 33: 1438–45.

10 Greer JA, Pirl WF, Jackson VA, *et al.* Effect of early palliative care on chemotherapy use and end-of-life care in patients with metastatic non-small-cell lung cancer. *J Clin Oncol* 2012; 30: 394–400.

11 van der Lee ML, van der Bom JG, Swarte NB, *et al.* Euthanasia and depression: a prospective cohort study among terminally ill cancer patients. *J Clin Oncol* 2005; 23: 6607–12.

12 Ruijs CD, van der Wal G, Kerkhof AJ, Onwuteaka-Philipsen BD. Unbearable suffering and requests for euthanasia prospectively studied in end-of-life cancer patients in primary care. *BMC Palliat Care* 2014; 13: 62.

13 Güell E, Ramos A, Zertuche T, Pascual A. Verbalized desire for death or euthanasia in advanced cancer patients receiving palliative care. *Palliat Support Care* 2015; 13: 295–303.

14 Suarez-Almazor ME, Newman C, Hanson J, Bruera E. Attitudes of terminally ill cancer patients about euthanasia and assisted suicide: predominance of psychosocial determinants and beliefs over symptom distress and subsequent survival. *J Clin Oncol* 2002; 20: 2134–41.

Further reading

* Department of Health (2008). *End of life care strategy. Promoting high quality care for all adults at the end of life.* Available from: www.gov.uk/government/uploads/system/uploads/attachment_data/file/136431/End_of_life_strategy.pdf (accessed 21 June 2017).

* Hansford P, Meehan H. Gold Standards Framework: improving community care. *End of Life Care* 2007; 1: 56–61.

* Macmillan Cancer Support (2012). *Preferred priorities for care document (England and Wales).* Available from: www.macmillan.org.uk/cancerinformation/livingwithandaftercancer/advancedcancer/advancecareplanning/englandandwales/preferredprioritiesforcaredocument.aspx (accessed 21 June 2017).

* National Confidential Enquiry into Patient Outcome and Death (2008). *For better, for worse? A review of the care of patients who died within 30 days of receiving systemic anti-cancer therapy.* Available from: www.ncepod.org.uk/2008report3/Downloads/SACT_report.pdf (accessed 21 June 2017).

* NHS Choices (2014). *Euthanasia and assisted suicide.* Available from: www.nhs.uk/conditions/Euthanasiaandassistedsuicide/Pages/Introduction.aspx (accessed 12 March 2017).

* NHS England (2016). *Enhanced supportive care: integrating supportive care in oncology. Phase I: treatment with palliative intent.* Available from: www.england.nhs.uk/wp-content/uploads/2016/03/ca1-enhncd-supprtv-care-guid.pdf (accessed 13 March 2017).

* Palumbo R, Sottotetti F, Riccardi A, *et al.* Which patients with metastatic breast cancer benefit from subsequent lines of treatment? An update for clinicians. *Ther Adv Med Oncol* 2013; 5: 334–50.

* Suicide Act 1961. Available from: www.legislation.gov.uk/ukpga/Eliz2/9-10/60 (accessed 12 March 2017).

05 Metastatic Adenocarcinoma of the Lung

Vinton Cheng, Denis Talbot

Case history

A 44-year-old man of Irish–Chinese descent with a diagnosis of metastatic epidermal growth factor receptor (EGFR)-positive adenocarcinoma of the lung was admitted to the acute oncology ward with severe vomiting during his initial cycle of first line palliative treatment with the tyrosine kinase inhibitor (TKI) gefitinib. It transpired that he had been taking traditional Chinese medicine alongside his treatment.

Following discussion with the oncology pharmacist he was given advice about potential interactions between traditional Chinese medicine and anticancer therapy. The medications were adapted and the patient continued his treatment without further incident.

How does improving cultural competence in cancer services enhance the patient experience and care received?

What communication issues may arise during a consultation with a patient from a black and minority ethnic group?

What impact can complementary and alternative medicine (CAM) have on oncological treatment?

What role could the multidisciplinary team (MDT) play in his cancer care?

How does improving cultural competence in cancer services enhance the patient experience and care received?

Cultural competence in the context of healthcare encompasses the behaviours, attitudes and actions of the individual healthcare professional and organizations that can help to manage potential conflict that may arise through differences in culture.[1] The definition of culture is far ranging and consists of the beliefs, behaviours, objectives and other characteristics common to members of a particular group or society. This case focuses on the role of ethnic background and language. It is important, however, for healthcare professionals to consider other factors that patients may use to define themselves, including sexuality, religion, geography, income and education.

We live in an increasingly diverse and multiethnic society. According to the 2011 census in England and Wales, over two decades the proportion of the population describing themselves as belonging to a black and minority ethnic group increased from 5.9% in 1991 to 14% in 2011.[2] As a result, coupled with a rising incidence of cancer,[3,4] more black and minority ethnic patients are engaging with cancer services across the UK. There is increasing concern about health inequalities in these groups, specifically access to cancer services, from screening to referral for specialist treatment to palliative and end-of-life care.[5,6] Promoting interactions and understanding between cancer care practitioners and black and minority ethnic patients may therefore significantly improve engagement with treatment and cancer outcomes.

The main impact of culture on healthcare arises from systematic health beliefs, rather than linguistic differences. Health beliefs relate to an internalized construct that informs an individual's understanding of health and illness. They may directly influence the patient's willingness to seek help when unwell, impact on the patient's description of symptoms and also affect adherence to treatment or follow-up. In Western societies, most healthcare professionals subscribe to the biomedical model. This explains disease in the context of biological processes; for example, lung cancer is known to be caused by genetic predisposition and environmental carcinogens such as tobacco smoking. By contrast, traditional Chinese health beliefs focus on maintaining balance and harmony, most notably through the concepts of *yin* and *yang*.[7] There is growing recognition that health is also influenced by social and psychological components; more recently, therefore, there has been greater acceptance of the biopsychosocial model proposed by Engel (Figure 5.1).[8]

The patient was clearly influenced by his ethnic background and upbringing in the way he approached his cancer treatment. A common mistake among healthcare practitioners is to view an acceptance of one set of health beliefs as a rejection of another. It is therefore possible to see

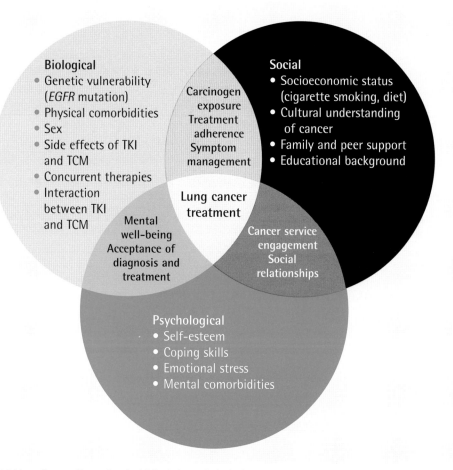

Figure 5.1 Venn diagram illustrating the biological, psychological and social determinants of the patient's lung cancer treatment according to the biopsychosocial model of health.[8] TCM, traditional Chinese medicine.

how his compliance with the TKI treatment might have resulted in the clinicians' oversight to enquire whether he was also taking any CAM therapies. From the perspective of the patient, there was no contradiction in accepting conventional treatment alongside traditional Chinese medicine, as according to his belief system both treatments were complementary in combating the cancer.

It is vital that cancer care practitioners take an active interest in their patients' backgrounds and cultural traditions. Fortunately, this predicament was handled sensitively and, rather than the patient's health beliefs being challenged, the healthcare system sought to accommodate his additional needs. This helped to establish a therapeutic relationship between the doctor and patient, resulting in not only improved treatment adherence but also enhanced patient satisfaction and clinical outcome.

What communication issues may arise during a consultation with a patient from a black and minority ethnic group?

The successful establishment of an effective doctor–patient relationship is underpinned by good communication. Cultural differences have the potential to undermine this relationship through language barriers and divergent beliefs. Language difficulties are known to be a key barrier to the engagement with cancer services of black and minority ethnic people.[9] The NHS has a wealth of resources to help tackle this issue, e.g. LanguageLine (www.languageline.com/uk), professional interpreters and translated documents. Despite the availability of resources, however, clinicians commonly rely on *ad hoc* family or staff interpreters due to perceived convenience of access. This has implications for communication with the patient, as these interpreters may lack training in medical terminology and may be less capable of acting as a cultural interface between the doctor and patient. The reliance on family members as interpreters also raises the risk of inadequate medical information being conveyed to the patient, as they might omit or filter important information in an attempt to shield their loved one.

In a recent study of breast cancer care it was shown that these communication difficulties negatively affected the ability of the clinician to provide patient-centred care and shared decision making, resulting in a paternalistic approach and simplification of the risk–benefit discussion.[10] This poses a particular challenge to the discussion around cancer treatment options such as surgery, radiotherapy and chemotherapy, where the significant risks need to be counterbalanced against the perceived benefits to the patient.

Although there were no language barriers with the patient, the cultural discordance manifested through an inadequate medication history during his initial consultation and subsequently upon admission to the acute oncology ward. It might have been possible to prevent admission to hospital or expedite recovery if the interaction with traditional Chinese medicine had been recognized earlier. Although clinicians can not be expected to have a full understanding of every patient's cultural background, this omission would have been easily prevented by thorough history taking, particularly focusing on the use of over-the-counter medications or CAM therapies.[11]

Another communication challenge that may arise during a consultation with a black and minority ethnic patient is when broaching potentially difficult topics such as cancer treatment goals and end-of-life care. Bekker's model, shown in Figure 5.2, highlights the complex interaction between the patient and the health professional during the consultation process, as each individual brings their own core attributes that include culture, experiences and personal views.[12,13] Cancer care practitioners must be willing to explore the added dimension of culture and acknowledge differing expressions of advanced disease and mortality. Only then may the doctor and patient reach a mutual understanding that will facilitate ongoing, shared decision making.

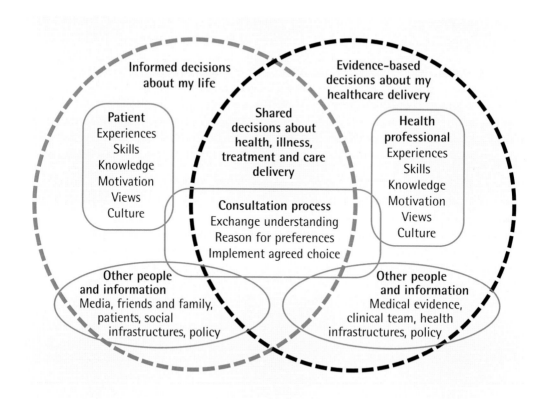

Figure 5.2 Bekker's model illustrating individual and collective decision making (adapted from Brown *et al.*[13]).

What impact can CAM have on oncological treatment?

CAM has been defined as 'a broad domain of healing resources that encompasses all health systems, modalities, and practices and their accompanying theories and beliefs, other than those intrinsic to the politically dominant health system of a particular society or culture in a given historical period'.[14] A review of cross-sectional surveys of adult cancer patients showed that a significant proportion (7–64%) use CAM therapies.[15] The wide variability in reported values is thought to be related to discrepancies in the understanding and definition of CAM therapies among healthcare professionals and patients.[15] It is also common for cancer patients to use CAM therapies while receiving conventional anticancer treatment,[16,17] as illustrated in our case.

The paucity of reliable evidence for CAM therapies, including traditional Chinese medicine, in the context of anticancer treatment has meant that its use is often viewed with suspicion and scepticism by healthcare professionals, as it contradicts their understanding of disease through the biopsychosocial model. If this conflict is outwardly manifested in their verbal or non-verbal communication it may negatively impact on the trust and communication between the clinician and the patient. It is possible that this patient chose not to tell the clinicians that he had been taking traditional Chinese medicine alongside gefitinib, due to perceived stigmatization. In this situation, he had been using extract of Gingko biloba, which has been shown to interact with TKIs by altering the action of the CYP3A4 isozyme.[18]

There is increasing recognition in Western medicine that CAM therapies can play a role as an adjunct to conventional cancer treatment, particularly for managing treatment-related side effects or for palliation of symptoms. Owing to this growing interest, active research is being undertaken to investigate the utility of specific CAM therapies, which may help to address some of the concerns of the healthcare profession. Acupuncture is one CAM therapy that is increasingly accepted in cancer services: it has been used for diverse functions including treating chemotherapy-induced nausea, cancer-associated fatigue, peripheral neuropathy and cancer-related pain. Although a large systematic review found that acupuncture may be effective as an adjunctive treatment for chemotherapy-induced nausea/vomiting, the overall poor quality of studies meant that further investigation was recommended.[19]

Despite healthcare professionals' anxiety around insufficient evidence, there is far less concern among the general public. One of the most appealing benefits of CAM therapy is the greater level of autonomy it affords the patient. At a time when patients may be suffering significant emotional distress and are psychologically at their most vulnerable, it would serve an empathetic clinician well to appreciate the impact distress may have on the patient's choices and modify the approach accordingly.

What role could the MDT play in his cancer care?

This case demonstrates the complex interaction between cancer services and a patient from a black and minority ethnic background. Along his journey the patient would have been in contact with multiple professionals from different disciplines and each one will have had an important role to play in the holistic management of his cancer. In this situation he would have particularly benefited from early intervention by the following nursing and allied health professionals:

- Clinical nurse specialists are registered nurses who have taken on a more specialist role in cancer care. They often fulfil diverse functions, but most importantly act as a key point of contact between the patient and the cancer service. Clinical nurse specialists can provide emotional support, alongside technical expertise, to help manage physical symptoms. Due to their significant contact time with the patient, they often have a thorough understanding of the individual's background and culture, which offers invaluable insight into how the patient may interact with the cancer service.[20]
- The oncology pharmacist provides access to expert resources on anticancer treatments, as well as an understanding of interactions with adjunctive and non-cancer therapies. In this case, the pharmacist played a key role in reconciling the medicines being taken by the patient and acted as an important interface in helping the doctor and patient to reach mutual understanding.
- In patients with nausea and vomiting, close monitoring of nutritional status and body mass is recommended. Ongoing support may be required from a specialist dietitian to monitor nutritional intake, particularly if modification of diet is part of CAM therapy.

Conclusion and learning points

- CAM therapies are often taken by patients without the knowledge of the treating clinician, which may impact on the doctor–patient relationship and lead to potential interaction with conventional treatments or reduced adherence to prescribed anticancer regimens.
- It is important that institutions promote greater understanding of CAM use among healthcare professionals and encourage them to discuss it with their patients.
- Cultural awareness and cultural competence are necessary skills for a satisfying and effective consultation, particularly with an increasingly diverse patient population.

- Adopting a non-judgemental approach and paying close attention to non-verbal communication will facilitate better communication with black and minority ethnic patients. If there are linguistic challenges, use of professional interpreters is recommended.

- The cancer MDT plays a pivotal role in ensuring the patient receives good-quality holistic care.

References

1 Surbone A. Cultural competence in oncology: where do we stand? *Ann Oncol* 2009; 21: 3–5.

2 Office for National Statistics (2012). *Ethnicity and national identity in England and Wales: 2011.* Available from: www.ons.gov.uk/peoplepopulationandcommunity/culturalidentity/ethnicity/articles/ethnicityandnationalidentityinenglandandwales/2012-12-11 (accessed 3 February 2017).

3 Smith LK, Botha JL, Benghiat A, *et al.* Latest trends in cancer incidence among UK South Asians in Leicester. *Br J Cancer* 2003; 89: 70–3.

4 Smith LK, Peake MD, Botha JL. Recent changes in lung cancer incidence for South Asians: a population based register study. *BMJ* 2003; 326: 8163.

5 Koffman J, Higginson IJ. Accounts of carers' satisfaction with health care at the end of life: a comparison of first generation black Caribbeans and white patients with advanced disease. *Palliat Med* 2001; 15: 337–45.

6 Thomas VN, Saleem T, Abraham R. Barriers to effective uptake of cancer screening among black and minority ethnic groups. *Int J Palliat Nurs* 2005; 11: 564–71.

7 Chen YC. Chinese values, health and nursing. *J Adv Nurs* 2001; 36: 270–3.

8 Engel G. The need for a new medical model: a challenge for biomedical science. *Science* 1977; 196: 126–9.

9 Abdullahi A, Copping J, Kessel A, *et al.* Cervical screening: perceptions and barriers to uptake among Somali women in Camden. *Public Health* 2009; 123: 680–5.

10 Karliner LS, Hwang ES, Nickleach D, *et al.* Language barriers and patient-centered breast cancer care. *Patient Educ Couns* 2011; 84: 223–8.

11 Cockayne NL, Duguid M, Shenfield GM. Health professionals rarely record history of complementary and alternative medicines. *Br J Clin Pharmacol* 2005; 59: 254–8.

12 Breckenridge K, Bekker HL, van der Veer SN, *et al.* How to routinely collect data on patient-reported outcome and experience measures in renal registries in Europe: an expert consensus meeting. *Nephrol Dial Transplant* 2015; 30: 1605–14.

13 Brown EA, Bekker HL, Davison SN, *et al.* Supportive care: communication strategies to improve cultural competence in shared decision making. *Clin J Am Soc Nephrol* 2016; 11: 1902–8.

14 Committee on the Use of Complementary and Alternative Medicine by the American Public, Board on Health Promotion and Disease Prevention, Institute of Medicine of the National Academies. *Complementary and alternative medicine in the United States.* Washington, DC: National Academies Press, 2005.

15 Ernst E, Cassileth BR. The prevalence of complementary/alternative medicine in cancer: a systematic review. *Cancer* 1998; 83: 777–82.

16 Downer SM, Cody MM, McCluskey P, *et al.* Pursuit and practice of complementary therapies by cancer patients receiving conventional treatment. *BMJ* 1994; 309: 86–9.

17 Crocetti E, Crotti N, Feltrin A, *et al.* The use of complementary therapies by breast cancer patients attending conventional treatment. *Eur J Cancer* 1998; 34: 324–8.

18 Yap KY, See CS, Chan A. Clinically-relevant chemotherapy interactions with complementary and alternative medicines in patients with cancer. *Recent Pat Food Nutr Agric* 2010; 2: 12–55.

19 Garcia MK, McQuade J, Haddad R, *et al.* Systematic review of acupuncture in cancer care: a synthesis of the evidence. *J Clin Oncol* 2013; 31: 952–60.

20 Department of Health National Cancer Action Team (2010). *Excellence in cancer care: the contribution of the clinical nurse specialist.* Available from: www.macmillan.org.uk/documents/aboutus/commissioners/ excellenceincancercarethecontributionoftheclinicalnursespecialist.pdf (accessed 3 February 2017).

Further reading

• Baccetti S, Di Stefano M, Di Vito M, *et al.* (2014). *Complementary and alternative medicine (CAM) in cancer care. Development and opportunities of integrative oncology.* Available from: www.epaac.eu/images/END/Final_Deliverables/D5_Complementary_and_alternative_ medicine_CAM_in_cancer_care_development_and_opportunities_of_integrative_oncology. pdf (accessed 12 February 2017).

• Redman J, Higginbottom GMA, Massey MT. Critical review of literature on ethnicity and health in relation to cancer and palliative care in the United Kingdom. *Divers Health Social Care* 2008; 5: 137–50.

• Wieland LS, Manheimer E, Berman BM. Development and classification of an operational definition of complementary and alternative medicine for the Cochrane collaboration. *Altern Ther Health Med* 2011; 17: 50–9.

06 Lessons Learnt from a Deaf Patient with Ovarian Cancer

Nicola Flaum, Jurjees Hasan

Case history

A 58-year-old woman with relapsed platinum-resistant high-grade serous carcinoma of the ovary was admitted with abdominal pain, distension and constipation. A CT scan showed multifocal small bowel obstruction from progressive peritoneal disease. At initial presentation she had International Federation of Gynecology and Obstetrics stage IIIC disease. She received surgery and adjuvant carboplatin and paclitaxel; after progression 8 months later she received another six cycles of carboplatin and paclitaxel, resulting in stable disease 6 weeks before admission. Her comorbidities included profound hearing loss since having meningitis as an infant. She lived with her husband, who was also deaf. She had chronic anxiety and worried about the impact of her disability on her treatment.

Options of chemotherapy and best supportive care were discussed through a British Sign Language (BSL) interpreter. Surgery to relieve bowel obstruction was not deemed feasible given diffuse serosal disease and multi-level small bowel obstruction. She wished to have chemotherapy, and commenced cisplatin and gemcitabine with parenteral nutritional support. Care was managed through a multidisciplinary team (MDT) comprising oncologists, palliative care specialists, specialist nurses, dietitians and a discharge planning team. A BSL interpreter was available every day to facilitate communication with the patient and her husband. Chemotherapy was withdrawn, as no clinical improvement was observed after two cycles of treatment. Following discussion with the patient and her family it was agreed she would go home and receive best supportive care. At the patient's request, a complex venting jejunostomy was fashioned to replace a nasogastric tube. Shortly afterwards, she developed intra-abdominal sepsis and died in hospital 9 weeks after admission.

What are the evidence base and rationale for this patient's treatment?

How did the patient's deafness affect her care?

How can communication in deaf cancer patients be optimized?

How do the principles of patient-centred care relate to this case?

What was the influence of integrated cancer care for this patient?

What are the evidence base and rationale for this patient's treatment?

Malignant bowel obstruction affects at least half of patients with ovarian cancer.[1] Cases with this complication are complex and require multidisciplinary input from oncologists, surgeons, the palliative care team, psycho-oncologists and dietitians. The prognosis, however, remains poor. A recent study found that the median overall survival in patients from diagnosis of bowel obstruction was 88 days;[2] therefore, management needs to be holistic and focused on balance in improving prognosis and symptom control with side effects of treatment.

The treatment of malignant bowel obstruction is largely best supportive care, focusing on symptom management and quality of life (QOL). In selected cases surgery and/or chemotherapy can be effective in managing symptoms, controlling disease and prolonging life.[2–5] The evidence base supporting chemotherapy is limited from retrospective case series. In one study of patients with malignant bowel obstruction, outcomes were not determined by platinum sensitivity. A simple prognostication tool based on performance status and type of obstruction (single- or multi-level) may be used in determining choice of therapy. This requires validation in a prospective study.

How did the patient's deafness affect her care?

Although the patient's medical management was unchanged, there were logistical considerations due to her deafness, as she required considerable input from the palliative care and symptom control team and other allied health professionals, necessitating a high degree of coordination with BSL interpreters. Quality of communication was a major issue for her and her family. Although it was acknowledged that it improved throughout admission, her family raised a complaint, 'to improve things for future deaf patients'. In addition to direct communication, interdisciplinary communication was important to her: that all staff knew her management plan and knew that she was deaf. Updating her and her family was made more challenging by BSL interpreters not being always available, which also affected her anxiety and its management.

She had a longstanding belief that she may be treated differently as a deaf patient, and was very sensitive to any perceived discrimination. For example, when told that the surgeons did not think surgery was the best option she stated this was because 'they didn't want to spend the money on me, [they think] I'm not worth saving'. Despite daily MDT review she stated she did not feel listened to or informed, although this improved throughout admission. A member of the palliative care and symptom control team described her attitude as a result of the inequalities she had faced as a deaf person and that she felt she had been treated differently from everyone else. She was very conscious of non-verbal behaviour and felt as if some of the staff were scared of her because of her deafness.

There is little research into mental health issues in the deaf community. Difficulty coping with communication and the psychosocial aspects of a hearing disability has been associated with higher anxiety levels in deaf patients undergoing physical rehabilitation.[6] A study of Norwegian deaf people found higher symptoms of depression and anxiety than in the general population.[7] A review of deaf patients' experience of the healthcare system reported that communication difficulties were ubiquitous, and that deaf patients frequently experienced fear, mistrust and frustration.[8] Deaf women have also been noted to experience barriers to accessing healthcare, to have limited knowledge of cancer prevention and screening, and to have significantly poorer knowledge of cancer generally and ovarian cancer specifically.[9] This can lead to greater communication challenges and affect how deaf patients view the healthcare system.

How can communication in deaf cancer patients be optimized?

It is important to be aware that deaf cancer patients might have had previous bad experiences in the healthcare system and have preconceived perceptions of healthcare professionals and medical treatment. It is vital to promote trust and build good professional relationships. Deaf patients have a legal right to request an interpreter, of which they may be unaware. It is best to avoid using relatives as interpreters, especially regarding complex decision making or bad news, as this can add additional distress for patients and their family. BSL interpreters are essential in optimizing communication and an interpreter should be arranged in coordination with clinical review, especially as regards giving results or decision making.

Communication can be optimized using multimodality methods and it is important to check deaf patients' literacy, writing ability and computer skills. Studies into communication of health and specifically cancer education in the deaf community have found that use of technology such as educational videos with a sign interpreter improved knowledge.[9] Many resources are available for deaf cancer patients. Macmillan Cancer Support provides BSL videos relating to chemotherapy, radiotherapy and surgery for cancer.[10] The deaf health charity SignHealth also provides information, BSL videos, community drop-in sessions and group sessions for deaf patients with a variety of health conditions including cancer, and runs awareness programmes such as ovarian cancer awareness month.[11] The British Deaf Association also offers information on communicating with deaf people and provides general support for the deaf community.

SignHealth advises optimizing awareness of patient needs to key workers, specialist nurses and the clinical team, and documenting this from the initial referral letter and MDT discussion. It should include the patient's communication method. Complex medical jargon should be avoided and, for patients who communicate by lip reading, consultations should take place in a well-lit room with minimum background noise for those with some residual hearing, hearing aids or cochlear implants. Maintain eye contact and ensure you have your patient's full attention before talking. Do not turn to face your computer while talking, look down to fill out paperwork or cover your mouth with your hands. Individualized care plans will be needed for management of patients on chemotherapy, including methods of communication at home for appointments and emergencies. Deafness should not be a barrier to clinical trial participation in eligible patients.[11]

How do the principles of patient–centred care relate to this case?

Patient-centred care incorporates the six domains of physical comfort: emotional support, respect for patients' preferences and values, integration and coordination, involvement of family and friends, communication, and education. As noted by Zucca et al.,[12] it is important for cancer centres to record and measure patient-centred care to allow for comparison and improvement. A BSL interpreter was booked and a clinical review arranged for the same time every day. Chemotherapy and intravenous medication were planned to be administered in the early morning, as the patient wished, which required close coordination between ward doctors, nurses, pharmacists and dietitians. It was important to the patient that the interpreter was always BSL trained and if possible was the same interpreter, including post-discharge in the community. After checking she understood the potential risks and benefits, patient preference was respected and she was given chemotherapy and a venting jejunostomy.

In this palliative situation the priority was QOL. While it is difficult to measure, the integration and coordination of the different allied health professionals were a significant focus of her care. The palliative care and symptom control team were involved from admission to assist in physical and emotional support, and the patient's family were also involved throughout. Communication and education were vital, as she did not have much pre-existing medical knowledge and had specific worries such as whether hugging her family had caused her infections.

What was the influence of integrated cancer care for this patient?

Many different hospital teams were involved in this patient's care, including the medical oncology team, ward junior doctors, nursing staff, palliative care and symptom control team, dietitians, community link/discharge team, patient advice and liaison service, interventional radiology, surgeons, and also ward clerks and administrative staff who were involved in coordinating care. Each team needed to liaise with the BSL interpreter service. In addition to inpatient teams the community teams are also vital for good, integrated care. Although the patient passed away before discharge, support was planned in the community through the community occupational therapists, her GP, BSL interpreters and the community link/discharge team. Considerations such as how we could communicate in an emergency were discussed, and text messaging was suggested for some emergency situations and a number given. This meant that she felt safer going home and it became more realistic and her priority.

Conclusion and learning points

- Advanced ovarian cancer frequently presents with malignant bowel obstruction, which needs to be managed in a multidisciplinary setting.
- The focus of treatment for advanced ovarian cancer is maintaining QOL and treating symptoms.
- Deaf patients experience more difficulty interacting with healthcare services and report feeling marginalized and disenfranchised by the healthcare system. Good communication involving sign interpreters is vital.
- Integrated patient-centred care is vital to optimize the care of cancer patients.

References

1 Pothuri B, Montemarano M, Gerardi M, et al. Percutaneous endoscopic gastrostomy tube placement in patients with malignant bowel obstruction due to ovarian carcinoma. *Gynecol Oncol* 2005; 96: 330–4.

2 Dean E, Khoja L, Clamp A, et al. Malignant bowel obstruction in advanced ovarian cancer. *Future Oncol* 2017; 13: 513–21.

3 Bryan DN, Radbod R, Berek JS. An analysis of surgical versus chemotherapeutic intervention for the management of intestinal obstruction in advanced ovarian cancer. *Int J Gynecol Cancer* 2006; 16: 125–34.

4 Kolomainen DF, Daponte A, Barton DP, et al. Outcomes of surgical management of bowel obstruction in relapsed epithelial ovarian cancer (EOC). *Gynecol Oncol* 2012; 125: 31–6.

5 Kucukmetin A, Naik R, Galaal K, et al. Palliative surgery versus medical management for bowel obstruction in ovarian cancer. *Cochrane Database Syst Rev* 2010; 7: CD007792.

6 Hogan A, Phillips RL, Brumby SA, et al. Higher social distress and lower psycho-social wellbeing: examining the coping capacity and health of people with hearing impairment. *Disabil Rehabil* 2015; 37: 2070–5.

7 Kvam MH, Loeb M, Tambs K. Mental health in deaf adults: symptoms of anxiety and depression among hearing and deaf individuals. *J Deaf Stud Educ* 2006; 12: 1–7.

8 Steinberg AG, Barnett S, Meador HE, et al. Health care system accessibility: experiences and perceptions of deaf people. *J Gen Intern Med* 2006; 21: 260–6.

9 Jensen LG, Nakaji M, Harry KM, et al. Ovarian cancer: deaf and hearing women's knowledge before and after an educational video. *J Cancer Educ* 2013; 28: 647–55.

10 Macmillan Cancer Support (2017). *British Sign Language (BSL) videos.* Available from:

www.macmillan.org.uk/information-and-support/resources-and-publications/other-formats/british-sign-language.html (accessed 20 January 2017).

11 SignHealth (2015). *March: ovarian cancer awareness month (BSL)*. Available from: www.signhealth.org.uk/march-ovarian-cancer-awareness-month-bsl (accessed 20 January 2017).

12 Zucca A, Sanson-Fisher R, Waller A, Carey M. Patient-centred care: making cancer treatment centres accountable. *Support Care Cancer* 2014; 22: 1989–97.

Further reading

- Ledermann JA, Kristeleit RS. Optimal treatment for relapsing ovarian cancer. *Ann Oncol* 2010; 21 (suppl 7): vii218–22.

07 A Young Man with Undiagnosed Autistic Spectrum Disorder and Hodgkin's Lymphoma

Alexandra R. Lewis, Kim Linton

Case history

A 23-year-old man presented with a 1 year history of neck lumps. He had refused to attend appointments for investigations but was eventually persuaded by his family to visit his GP.

He was diagnosed with stage IIA Hodgkin's lymphoma, with no unfavourable features, and referred for consideration of treatment with chemotherapy +/− radiotherapy. The patient attended with his father, aunt and grandmother but not his mother, with whom he was living. He was awaiting an appointment to undergo testing for Asperger's syndrome. His family stated that he was very intelligent. He appeared to interpret speech very literally and it was difficult to tell whether he fully comprehended the information given.

Two doctors agreed that he had capacity to consent for chemotherapy, and he gave signed, informed consent to treatment with doxorubicin, bleomycin, vinblastine and dacarbazine (ABVD). Three cycles were planned followed by a PET-CT scan to guide the need for further therapy based on the response to chemotherapy.

A diagnosis of autistic spectrum disorder was confirmed during treatment, when it also became apparent that relations between the patient and his mother had broken down. Consequently, his mother tried to access information about his diagnosis directly from staff. He was assigned a social worker from the young-oncology service to support him during treatment. As he became very distressed waiting for consultations in waiting rooms, arrangements were made for him to wait for clinic appointments in the teen and young adult lounge instead.

As treatment continued, the patient's mental state deteriorated and he was referred to the psycho-oncology service. He was reviewed by a clinical psychologist and diagnosed with an anxiety disorder. His family were referred to points of support such as the National Autistic Society, and strategies for managing anxiety were discussed with his key worker.

The patient completed three cycles of ABVD chemotherapy without significant toxicity; a repeat PET scan showed a complete metabolic response. As he did not require further chemotherapy or radiotherapy, he entered post-treatment surveillance.

What were the aims of treatment for this patient?

What is the evidence base for the treatment?

What is autistic spectrum disorder and how did it affect the patient's treatment?

What issues need to be considered when treating patients with autistic spectrum disorder who are undergoing treatment in the oncology department?

What were the aims of treatment for this patient?

With modern combined modality treatment (chemotherapy and radiotherapy), patients with Hodgkin's lymphoma stage I/II disease and no adverse risk factors achieve 5 year survival rates exceeding 90%.[1] The aim of treatment in our patient was to cure the disease using the minimum amount of treatment and disruption given his concomitant diagnosis of Asperger's syndrome and fractured social background.

What is the evidence base for the treatment?

Early-stage Hodgkin's lymphoma was historically treated with radiotherapy alone. The German Hodgkin Study Group, however, demonstrated a considerable reduction in relapse rates when two cycles of ABVD chemotherapy were added to extended-field radiotherapy (GHSG HD7 trial).[2] The freedom from treatment failure rate in the arm treated with ABVD plus radiotherapy was 88% at 7 years compared with 67% in those treated with radiotherapy alone. This led to a change in practice. More recently, the GHSG HD10 trial confirmed that two cycles of ABVD followed by low-dose radiotherapy (20 Gy involved-field radiation) is as effective as, and less toxic than, four cycles of ABVD followed by 30 Gy involved-field radiation.[3] There is, however, strong evidence that the use of radiotherapy increases the risk of a secondary solid malignancy, notably cancers of the breast and lung in patients treated with supradiaphragmatic fields. A recent Dutch study assessed the incidence of second cancers after treatment for Hodgkin's lymphoma in patients treated between 1965 and 2000.[4] It compared those treated between 1965 and 1989 with those treated between 1989 and 2000, when modern treatment with smaller radiotherapy doses and fields, less infradiaphragmatic radiotherapy and more anthracycline-based chemotherapy was introduced. The study reported a cumulative incidence of second cancers of 33.2% at 30 years after the start of treatment for Hodgkin's lymphoma compared with 9.6% for the general population. When comparing the two time periods, there was no significant difference in the cumulative incidence of second solid cancers. Thus, a risk of second cancers remains high in the modern treatment era and, since risks increase with radiotherapy dose and time since treatment, the desire to avoid radiotherapy is greatest in young, cured patients. A large randomized phase III National Cancer Research Network trial, A Randomized Phase III Trial to Determine the Role of FDG-PET Imaging in Clinical Stages IA/IIA Hodgkin's Disease (RAPID), addressed the impact of avoiding radiotherapy in patients with a high chance of being cured by chemotherapy alone.[5] Patients with non-bulky early-stage Hodgkin's lymphoma and a negative PET-CT scan after three cycles of ABVD, i.e. complete metabolic response indicating no residual disease, were randomized to receive radiotherapy or no further treatment after chemotherapy. Omitting radiotherapy in this favourable prognostic group produced a slightly inferior 3 year progression-free survival of 90.8% compared with 94.6% in the standard ABVD plus radiotherapy arm. Longer follow-up is needed to assess the impact on overall survival, and in particular whether it is offset by a reduction in second cancers. Results of the RAPID trial nevertheless show that it is possible to achieve excellent outcomes in PET-negative patients without the addition of radiotherapy, thereby providing choice in patients in whom radiotherapy is undesirable. This was the case for our patient, as further treatment was not in his best interest because of his deteriorating mental state.

What is autistic spectrum disorder and how did it affect the patient's treatment?

Autistic spectrum disorder is a pervasive neurodevelopmental disorder characterized by speech and social communication difficulties and restricted and repetitive behaviour patterns.[6] It is commonly associated with other conditions including attention deficit disorder, abnormal responsiveness to sensory stimuli, and aggressive behaviours. As indicated by the term spectrum it comprises a very heterogeneous patient group (including individuals with Asperger's syndrome), and the degree of social and educational functioning can vary widely. For example, speech can range from the patient being entirely non-verbal to having relatively normal communication but with a tendency to interpret speech very literally and to struggle with language expressions such as sarcasm. Our patient presented with these features and it was challenging for treating physicians to assess his level of understanding.

The patient presented with symptoms of anxiety and his family reported aggressive behaviour. Engagement with his family was vital to ensuring that he completed treatment in a timely fashion. The patient would rarely open mail; therefore, his key worker had to phone him to inform him of appointments. His family would also be informed so that he could be encouraged to attend.

Because of sensory overload he found busy clinic waiting rooms stressful, and this was helped by arrangements for him to wait in the teen and young adult lounge where distractions (such as TV and games) were available. This reduced his stress levels and improved treatment compliance. We also moved appointments to allow him to attend his apprenticeship, as he found missing work distressing.

Involvement of the psycho-oncology service was useful in providing support to his family and advice in managing his symptoms. The family were also supported by charities such as the National Autistic Society.

What issues need to be considered when treating patients with autistic spectrum disorder who are undergoing treatment in the oncology department?

Oncology care requires a high level of commitment from the patient. Regular appointments, frequently invasive tests and delivery of treatment require organization and are significantly disruptive to daily life. These can be difficult to countenance for any patient. Advice for health professionals is available from the National Autistic Society.[7]

- Patients with autistic spectrum disorder should be provided with all the resources necessary to give informed consent. This may require the use of different resources, e.g. pictures, and significantly more time to discuss information.
- Because of sensory overload in many patients with autistic spectrum disorder, it may be necessary to allow the patient to await appointments in a quiet area. Similarly, an early or late appointment may minimize waiting times.
- Patients with autistic spectrum disorder may interpret speech very literally: staff should avoid using euphemisms and use direct instructions, e.g. 'stretch out your arm' rather than 'can you show me your arm'.

- Patients may not offer information and staff may need to use direct questioning.
- It may be useful to show patients around the treatment centre and allow them to see others undergoing treatment to prepare them for what to expect.
- A cancer diagnosis is a stressful time. The effects of this stress may be demonstrated differently in a patient with autistic spectrum disorder, for example in altered behaviour or repetitive physical mannerisms.
- The patient's carers will have the best knowledge of the patient's particular needs and must be involved in decision making. Care should be undertaken by a multidisciplinary team (MDT), involving the patient where possible, as well as the patient's caregivers, a key worker from the teen and young adult or learning disability teams, and other health professionals.
- Capacity to give informed consent must be assessed according to the Mental Capacity Act 2005. If the patient lacks capacity then consent for treatment can be given by proxy in the patient's best interests. The Mental Capacity Act advises that the least restrictive treatment be given.

Conclusion and learning points

- Patients with autistic spectrum disorder or other neurodevelopmental disorders undergoing cancer treatment are likely to require adjustments to treatment plans in accordance with their individual needs.
- Involvement of carers is vital to guide care needs and ensure treatment compliance.
- With the involvement of the MDT, it is possible to deliver timely care with minimal disruption and the expectation of similar clinical outcomes to those of patients treated without autistic spectrum disorder.

References

1 Eichenauer DA, Engert A, Andre M, *et al.* Hodgkin's lymphoma: ESMO clinical practice guidelines for diagnosis, treatment and follow-up. *Ann Oncol* 2014; 25 (suppl 3): 70–5.

2 Engert A, Franklin J, Eich HT, *et al.* Two cycles of doxorubicin, bleomycin, vinblastine and dacarbazine plus extended-field radiotherapy is superior to radiotherapy alone in early favourable Hodgkin's lymphoma: final results of the GHSG HD7 trial. *J Clin Oncol* 2007; 25: 3495–502.

3 Engert A, Plutschow A, Eich HT, *et al.* Reduced treatment intensity in patients with early-stage Hodgkin's lymphoma. *N Engl J Med* 2010; 363: 640–52.

4 Schaapveld M, Aleman BMP, van Eggermond AM, *et al.* Second cancer risk up to 40 years after treatment for Hodgkin's lymphoma. *N Engl J Med* 2015; 373: 2499–511.

5 Radford J, Illidge T, Counsell N, *et al.* Results of a trial of PET-directed therapy for early-stage Hodgkin's lymphoma. *N Engl J Med* 2015; 372: 1598–607.

6 National Institute for Health and Care Excellence (2012). *Autism spectrum disorder in adults: diagnosis and management. Clinical guideline CG142.* Available from: nice.org.uk/guidance/cg142 (accessed 1 March 2017).

7 National Autistic Society. *Health and social care workers.* Available from: www.autism.org.uk/professionals/health-workers.aspx (accessed 1 March 2017).

Further reading

- NHS Protect. *Meeting needs and reducing distress. Guidance on the prevention and management of clinically related challenging behaviour in NHS settings.* Available from: www.reducingdistress.co.uk/reducingdistress (accessed 1 March 2017).

08 A T3N1 Oesophageal Adenocarcinoma Patient Refusing Curative Surgery for Seemingly Irrational Reasons

Maung Maung Myat Moe, Clare Kane, Cate Simmons, Lucinda Melcher

Case history

A 69-year-old man presented with a short history of dysphagia. His medical history included a leg angioplasty, hypercholesterolaemia and atrial fibrillation. He took clopidogrel, rivaroxaban and gabapentin. He was a smoker and a moderate drinker, and ran a busy domestic cleaning service. Investigations confirmed moderately differentiated invasive adenocarcinoma of the oesophagus on a background of Barrett's oesophagus. CT staging was T3N1M0. The upper gastrointestinal multidisciplinary team (MDT) recommended neoadjuvant chemotherapy followed by curative surgery.

The patient attended the medical oncology clinic with his wife to go through the treatment plan. As ours is a cancer unit in a district general hospital, only chemotherapy is given locally and the surgery is performed in a tertiary care centre in central London. Radiotherapy is given in a cancer centre about 25 miles away.

Despite a good chance of cure, he declined the plan with surgery because he did not like going to central London. He also refused to go to other centres because of the distance. He wanted to take only chemotherapy that was given locally. Definitive chemoradiotherapy (dCRT) was offered as an alternative for a better result. After knowing the duration and daily commuting for radiotherapy, chemotherapy schedules and potential side effects, he declined all treatments because he was concerned that he would not be able to serve his customers due to the time commitment and side effects. He denied financial reasons for his decision. Although it was made explicit to him that he could die prematurely from this cancer if left untreated, he was adamant that he did not want to miss serving his customers and preferred to let 'what will be will be'. His wife, the clinical nurse specialist and the consultant all agreed that he had full mental capacity and understood the seriousness of the condition and the consequences of not having treatments.

The clinical nurse specialist continued supporting him by phone. Two weeks later, as his dysphagia got slightly worse, he agreed, and eventually took, a full course of chemoradiotherapy (50 Gy in 25 fractions, with weekly carboplatin and paclitaxel). A PET-CT scan done at 12 weeks after completion of the treatment showed no definite recurrence.

What could be done if he continues refusing treatment?

By not having the curative surgical approach recommended by the MDT, how
could his prognosis be affected?

How should he be followed up for best outcome taking into account his
commitment to his work?

What could be done if he continues refusing treatment?

Some patients make decisions about a treatment based on their personal values, experience and
circumstances rather than the side effects and benefits of treatment.[1] The General Medical
Council's guidance is to respect a competent patient's decision to refuse a treatment even if it
seems to be wrong or irrational to others. Anything that may imply judgement of a patient or of
his/her beliefs and values should be avoided. The patient may be provided with clinical opinions
but no pressure should be exerted to have the decision changed, otherwise this could lead to the
patient not feeling free to make his/her own decision, as well as to frustration, miscommunication
and a poor doctor–patient relationship, possibly resulting in refusal to have any future contact
with healthcare professionals.[2,3]

According to the Mental Capacity Act 2005 any person over age 16 is assumed to have mental
capacity unless it is established that s/he lacks capacity. The professional responsible for the
treatment and directly concerned with the individual at the time has to assess the capacity. An
interactive online tool to assist doctors in assessing a patient's capacity has been recently made
available on the General Medical Council website.[4] The first step is to maximize capacity by giving
treatment options (and information that includes the consequences of deciding one way or another
or of failing to take the treatment) at a suitable time and place, in the presence of friends, family
and other healthcare team members, using the most appropriate ways of communication such as
audio recording, printed information, etc. In a second step, the patient's abilities to understand,
retain and weigh up the given information and communicate his or her wishes should be assessed.
Without these, the patient lacks capacity to make the decision, in which case the patient's advance
wishes, or any wishes of which friends and relatives are aware, should be explored and acted upon
in the best interest of the patient. In the absence of these, an application to the court can be made
for someone with lasting power of attorney, or a court-appointed deputy or independent mental
capacity advocate, to represent the patient to make the decision.

As our patient had full mental capacity, as assessed by two medical professionals and his wife at
the time of making the decision, his decision should be fully respected. He should be offered full
support, which he was, and quick and full medical care if he changes his mind in the future.

By not having the curative surgical approach recommended by the MDT, how could his prognosis be affected?

Current standard treatment for T3N1 oesophageal adenocarcinoma in a medically fit patient is
neoadjuvant chemotherapy/chemoradiotherapy followed by surgery. There are no randomized
trial data to evaluate the difference in survival between having and not having surgery.

In the Neoadjuvant Chemoradiation Followed by Surgery versus Surgery Alone for Patients with
Adenocarcinomas or Squamous Cell Carcinomas of the Esophagus (CROSS) trial,[5] after a median
follow-up of 84.1 months for surviving patients (range 61.1–116.8 months), median overall
survival for adenocarcinoma patients treated with concurrent chemoradiotherapy (weekly
carboplatin AUC 2 and paclitaxel 50 mg/m^2 for 5 weeks) followed by surgery was 43.2 months
(95% CI 24.9, 61.4) and 27.1 months (95% CI 13.0, 41.2) for surgery only. The extra survival gain
of 16 months suggests a significant impact of the chemoradiotherapy component. The pathological

complete response (pCR) rate to chemoradiotherapy was 29%. A phase II study using the same chemoradiotherapy followed by surgery (75% of participants with adenocarcinoma) reported a pCR rate of 25%.[6] No survival difference was found between patients with or without pCR, suggesting surgery may be beneficial only to those who failed to achieve pCR.

A single centre retrospective study using propensity score analysis showed identical median and 2 year rates for disease-free (10 months, 33.8%) and overall survival (23 months, 47.3%) for stage III patients in both cohorts of 244 dCRT patients (patient's choice 14%; adenocarcinoma 55.3%; T3 59.8%; N1 62.3%) and 277 surgery patients, with or without neoadjuvant chemotherapy/chemoradiotherapy (adenocarcinoma 80.9%; T3 67.9%; N1 53.4%).[7]

A recent Cochrane review did not find any statistically significant difference in long-term survival between dCRT and neoadjuvant chemotherapy/chemoradiotherapy followed by surgery, whether analysed as a binary outcome (RR 1.04; 95% CI 0.93, 1.16; 431 participants) or as a time-to-event outcome (HR 0.99; 95% CI 0.78, 1.26; 431 participants).[8] However, owing to the small number of patients, the review could not rule out significant benefits or harms of dCRT versus surgery for adenocarcinoma.

dCRT using either fluorouracil, folinic acid and oxaliplatin (FOLFOX) or cisplatin and fluorouracil in 267 patients (stage III 57%; adenocarcinoma 14%; surgery unsuitable 74%) gave median progression-free survival of 9.55 months for the whole cohort, and median overall survival for stages I–III disease of 23.5 months using FOLFOX chemotherapy and 17.4 months using cisplatin and fluorouracil.[9]

In SCOPE 1, a trial that used cisplatin and capecitabine with or without cetuximab concurrently according to a very strict radiotherapy protocol, patients with no residual cancer on endoscopic biopsy and CT scan carried out 12 weeks after completion of the dCRT achieved median overall survival of 26.7 months (stage III 60%; adenocarcinoma 25%).[10]

Based on the available evidence, we can not confidently rule out any detrimental impact on our patient's survival by not having surgery, although it may be small if he achieves pCR from dCRT.

How should he be followed up for best outcome taking into account his commitment to his work?

Routine follow-up involves clinic reviews every 3–4 months for 2 years and yearly thereafter, and further endoscopy and a CT scan if symptoms occur. If he does not want to make regular visits because of his work commitments, it would be reasonable to ask him to agree to get in touch with the team as soon as he notices a new symptom. This will be more appropriate for him, especially if endoscopic biopsy and a CT scan 12 weeks after treatment do not show any evidence of disease.

Loco-regional recurrence is more common in dCRT patients compared with surgery patients.[7] According to a Cochrane review, patients receiving dCRT are also more likely to suffer from dysphagia in the later stage of the disease compared with those who undergo surgery (RR 1.48; 95% CI 1.01, 2.19; 139 participants; one study; very low-quality evidence).[8] Thorough endoscopic biopsy and CT examination are vital to differentiate between local recurrence and radiotherapy-induced oesophageal stricture. Salvage surgery can be offered for localized recurrence. Surgery can also be useful for radiation-induced stricture when other measures fail. Despite his current refusal of a surgical option, he might change his mind in the future for various reasons, and the opportunity should be made available to him for a quick assessment at first development of dysphagia or other symptoms. If he loses his mental capacity in the future, however, his decision for no surgery should be respected unless he makes someone aware of a change of mind while he has full capacity. Palliative chemotherapies could also be offered for metastatic disease for a small survival benefit.

Occasional follow-up telephone calls by the clinical nurse specialist, choosing a specific time outside his working hours, could make him more willing to seek help at the earliest opportunity. Any concerns about finance should be addressed and advice given.

Conclusion and learning points

- Every person over age 16 is assumed to have capacity to make decisions unless proven otherwise.

- A person lacks capacity to make a decision if s/he is unable to understand, retain or weigh the given information or communicate the decision to others.

- A competent person's decision to refuse treatment should be respected no matter how wrong or irrational it may seem to others; continuing support should be given to maintain a good relationship and encourage the patient to come back when help is needed.

- Anything that may imply judgement of a patient or of his/her beliefs and values should be avoided.

- There is no high-quality evidence to evaluate the survival difference between definitive chemoradiotherapy and neoadjuvant chemotherapy/chemoradiotherapy followed by curative surgery for operable stages I–III oesophageal adenocarcinoma in medically fit patients.

- A median survival of 43.2 months in adenocarcinoma patients treated with carboplatin and paclitaxel, and concurrent radiotherapy followed by surgery, in the CROSS trial is the best treatment outcome to date.

- Loco-regional recurrence and dysphagia in a later stage occur more commonly in dCRT patients compared with surgery patients.

References

1   van Kleffens T, van Leeuwen E. Physicians' evaluations of patients' decisions to refuse oncological treatment. *J Med Ethics* 2005; 31: 131–6.

2   van Kleffens T, van Baarsen B, van Leeuwen E. The medical practice of patient autonomy and cancer treatment refusals: a patients' and physicians' perspective. *Soc Sci Med* 2004; 58: 2325–36.

3   General Medical Council (2013). *Personal beliefs and medical practice.* Available from: www.gmc-uk.org/guidance/ethical_guidance/21171.asp (accessed 13 February 2017).

4   General Medical Council (2017). *Decision making when patients may lack capacity.* Available from: www.gmc-uk.org/Mental_Capacity_flowchart (accessed 26 January 2017).

5   Shapiro J, van Lanschot JJ, Hulshof MC, *et al.* Neoadjuvant chemoradiotherapy plus surgery versus surgery alone for oesophageal or junctional cancer (CROSS): long-term results of a randomised controlled trial. *Lancet Oncol* 2015; 16: 1090–8.

6   van Meerten E, Muller K, Tilanus HW, *et al.* Neoadjuvant concurrent chemoradiation with weekly paclitaxel and carboplatin for patients with oesophageal cancer: a phase II study. *Br J Cancer* 2006; 94: 1389–94.

7   Karran A, Blake P, Chan D, *et al.* Propensity score analysis of oesophageal cancer treatment with surgery or definitive chemoradiotherapy. *Br J Surg* 2014; 101: 502–10.

8 Best LM, Mughal M, Gurusamy KS. Non-surgical versus surgical treatment for oesophageal cancer. *Cochrane Database Syst Rev* 2016; 3: CD011498.

9 Conroy T, Galais MP, Raoul JL, *et al.* Definitive chemoradiotherapy with FOLFOX versus fluorouracil and cisplatin in patients with oesophageal cancer (PRODIGE5/ACCORD17): final results of a randomised, phase 2/3 trial. *Lancet Oncol* 2014; 15: 305–14.

10 Crosby T, Hurt C, Falk S, *et al.* Chemoradiotherapy with or without cetuximab in patients with oesophageal cancer (SCOPE 1): a multicentre, phase 2/3 randomised trial. *Lancet Oncol* 2013; 14: 627–37.

Further reading

* Mental Capacity Act 2005. Available from: www.legislation.gov.uk/ukpga/2005/9/pdfs/ukpga_20050009_en.pdf (accessed 13 February 2017).

09 A Patient with Brain Cancer: from Diagnosis to Treatment

Yin Zhou

Case history

 A 56-year-old woman presented to her GP with a 10 day history of frontal headache in the context of orthodontic work. She then developed mild confusion and left facial droop over a 3 week period. On her third GP visit, she was referred to the emergency outpatient neurology clinic (normally seen within days), after discussion with the neurologist on call. During the weekend, she was referred to A&E by an out-of-hours GP, with worsening symptoms. She was diagnosed with frontal lobe glioblastoma and underwent surgery, chemotherapy and radiotherapy. The overall treatment intent was palliation and symptom control.

After hospital discharge, a follow-up GP appointment was scheduled to explore her understanding of the diagnosis, prognosis and treatment plan. She had one daughter of early adult age and a husband with multiple sclerosis who lived in a nursing home. She was issued a Med 3 fit note (i.e. sickness certificate) for 2 months initially and encouraged to explore her employment options with her employer.

A lead GP was assigned to the patient, who was also added to the practice multidisciplinary team (MDT) discussion list. Active cancer treatment was promptly communicated to primary care through frequent clinic letters. She responded well to the chemoradiotherapy and had no recurrence until 16 months after diagnosis. When disease progressed, the neuro-oncology MDT team decided that it was not in her best interest to undergo further systemic therapies due to bone marrow suppression from the second line chemotherapy.

The decision to stop all treatments came as a shock to the patient, who had had 16 months of relatively normal life. She was referred to the local hospice. She was visited and supported by the palliative care nurse, who explored the patient's worries about her only daughter (who was at university), assisted with applying for disability allowance (form DS1500) and provided regular updates during the monthly practice MDT meeting. A lasting power of attorney was set up. Joint home visits with the GP and palliative care nurse were arranged. Dosette boxes and twice daily social care were arranged, while input from the occupational therapist and district nurses was also sought.

In the subsequent 2 months, the patient developed a head droop and shuffling gait. A do-not-resuscitate order was signed after discussion with her and her health and welfare attorney. 'Just-in-case' medications were delivered. She was subsequently admitted to the hospice for symptom control, following two focal seizures and increased agitation, and passed away peacefully a month later.

How did the patient's presentation affect her diagnostic pathway and time to diagnosis?

What was the role of her GP in providing patient-centred care?

What were the roles of the palliative care services in providing holistic and integrated care?

How did integrated care play a part in the management plan?

How did the patient's presentation affect her diagnostic pathway and time to diagnosis?

In the UK, the majority of symptomatic cancer patients first present to primary care. Strategies to improve early diagnosis have been a major focus of research and policy interventions in recent years. In judging whether diagnosis was timely, it is important to consider whether there were any missed opportunities for more optimal care during the diagnostic process.

Organizational factors

Access to routine and out-of-hours primary care, and to emergency and urgent specialist care (including 2-week-wait fast-track clinics), allows prompt assessment of symptomatic patients with possible cancer. Our patient was referred to the emergency neurology clinic after the third presentation to her GP, which represented the fastest non-emergency route to obtaining a neurological review locally. Access to 24/7 primary care allowed prompt reassessment of developing symptoms and signs. Sharing of in-hours and out-of-hours GP records also facilitated informational continuity of care in this case.

Patient factors

Prompt reappraisal of symptoms was facilitated by specific safety netting advice from her GP, enabling her to seek help quickly when her symptoms did not fit the expected nature of progression.

Biological factors

Brain cancer has one of the lowest 2-week-wait referral rates among all cancers due to its non-specific presenting symptoms and rarity. The rapid progression of symptoms over a 3 week period, combined with prompt symptom appraisal and good access to healthcare, allowed a relatively timely diagnosis within currently available resources.

What was the role of her GP in providing patient-centred care?

Her GP was instrumental in providing care at each of the following stages from first presentation to treatments.

Diagnosis

Her GP played a crucial role in clinical diagnosis, safety netting and engaging help from relevant allied health professionals (such as physiotherapist and occupational therapist). Out-of-hours GPs may act as a first point of contact for emergency presenters during evenings and weekends.

At and after diagnosis

A prompt follow-up GP appointment was arranged after the patient's discharge from hospital (within days). It was important to establish her level of understanding of the diagnosis, prognosis and treatment, and to identify her concerns and worries. It is important for GPs to understand the level of social support (both formal and informal) available to the patient and the individual responsibilities (employment, dependants) of the patient, in order to identify future and unmet needs that should be addressed.

During active treatment
Patients undergoing chemo- and radiotherapy often experience side effects from treatments. Although these patients usually have direct access to specialist oncology teams during working hours, they may still present to GPs both in- and out-of-hours.

End-of-life phase
Do-not-resuscitate decisions and a lasting power of attorney were discussed and set up in advance in primary care. Medications for palliative symptoms such as pain, secretions, agitation and nausea were also prepared in good time after discussion with the patient and family.

Care coordination
GPs play a key role in identifying patients who may need palliative care, so that advance care planning can commence as soon as possible. Most GP surgeries will have a list of vulnerable patients and palliative care patients for regular MDT discussions, although there are variations in the scope and delivery of MDTs between practices across the UK. Palliative care patients are actively identified using tools such as the Gold Standards Framework (www.goldstandardsframework.org.uk),[1] which recommends active care planning. Health professionals from the rest of the community, including district nurses, community matron, palliative care team, community psychiatric nurse, physiotherapist and occupational therapist, may attend. Some of these MDT lists are managed by MDT coordinators who help serve as a point of contact for patients and carers when they have difficulty navigating between different members of the MDT.

What were the roles of the palliative care services in providing holistic and integrated care?

The scope of palliative care services varies from providing inpatient services and day therapy units to hospice care at home. Other specialist services may include providing complementary therapy, patient and family support, and education to the public and professionals.

The palliative care nurse was able to do the following:

- Manage symptoms through medical and non-pharmacological methods.
- Provide psychosocial support for the patient and her daughter, addressing their concerns while respecting their wishes and preferences.
- Initiate and ensure future care planning such as supporting the application for government benefits (the DS1500 form is a personal independence payment issued for people aged 16–64 with a terminal disease and life expectancy of 6 months or less).
- Ensure integrated care by facilitating communication between the palliative care MDT, GP, district nurses and wider community, including physiotherapists and district nurse, enabling complex decision making and end-of-life planning.

How did integrated care play a part in the management plan?

Integrated care can occur at the macro, meso or micro level;[2] the majority of integrated care in the UK is performed at the micro level. NHS England states that integration of health, care and support 'must be person-centred, coordinated, and tailored to the needs and preferences of the individual, the individual's carer and the family'.[3]

- Macro level: providers and commissioners deliver primary and specialist services to the populations they serve (common in the USA).
- Meso level: integrated care delivered for patient subgroups through programmes or clinical networks.
- Micro level: care is delivered for individual patients and their family through active care coordination.

During the active treatment period, timely communication between primary care and the neuro-oncologists is paramount. Clinic letters were sent to the practice within days, and follow-up plans were promptly and clearly communicated to the GP. Blood tests performed in primary care were sent to the hospital and were therefore accessible by the specialists. The GPs also had direct access to the oncology team via the oncology nurses during working hours, or the on-call oncology team out-of-hours, so that information, clarification and advice could be sought from secondary care. In the community, regular MDT meetings at the GP practice allow the wider MDT to be kept informed of the various aspects of care and to carry out active care planning. Active case management by a member of the MDT is essential to facilitate integrated care.

Integration of primary care, oncology and palliative care services should occur early and throughout the diagnostic and treatment journey of cancer patients. Conceptual models of integration between the three services have been described in the following ways:[4]

- Time-based model: relevant services are involved as the need arises along the disease trajectory.
- Provider-based model: involvement of relevant palliative care services according to patient complexity and setting (i.e. escalation from primary to secondary to tertiary care).
- Issue-based model: integration based mainly on clinical need.
- System-based model: complements the issue-based model, where integration of services occurs when a patient meets the predefined criteria (but including all biopsychosocial factors).

In particular, the integrated system-based model advocates a patient-centred approach in which all biopsychosocial factors of the patient and family are considered, and relevant services are involved in a holistic way to enable shared decision making.

Conclusion and learning points

- Integrated care between specialists, GPs and the wider community should aim to address the clinical, psychological and social needs of the patient.
- Access to, and prompt communication among, all involved teams is crucial in enabling informational and relational continuity of care for cancer patients. System changes such as the sharing of primary care (in-hours and out-of-hours) and specialist care records will facilitate such continuity.
- Active case management (by the GP, MDT coordinator or the palliative care nurse) is important in providing integrated cancer care.

- Future integration should not only merge services but also aim to bring together commissioners and providers so that incentives can be aligned (integration at the macro level).

References

1 Gómez-Batiste X, Murray SA, Thomas K, *et al.* Comprehensive and integrated palliative care for people with advanced chronic conditions: an update from several European initiatives and recommendations for policy. *J Pain Symptom Manage* 2017; 53: 509–17.

2 Ham C, Curry N. *Integrated care. What is it? Does it work? What does it mean for the NHS?* London: The King's Fund, 2011.

3 NHS England (2013). *Integrated care and support.* Available from: www.england.nhs.uk/ourwork/part-rel/transformation-fund (accessed 1 April 2017).

4 Hui D, Bruera E. Models of integration of oncology and palliative care. *Ann Palliat Med* 2015; 4: 89–98.

10 A Woman Presenting to Primary Care with Painful Bone Metastases

Lucy Flanders, Mulyati Mohamed, Pauline Leonard

Case history

 A 69-year-old woman presented to her GP with a 2 month history of increasing back pain. She had no significant medical history. Her GP referred her for X-rays of her thoracic and lumbar spine. The reporting radiologist recommended a whole spine MRI scan, as sclerotic abnormalities were identified in the L1 and L4 vertebrae. An MRI requested by her GP was performed within 10 days and confirmed the presence of multiple bone metastases but no evidence of malignant spinal cord compression. The reporting radiologist contacted the acute oncology team by email and added the contact details of the acute oncology service on the bottom of the report for the GP to follow up.

The patient was seen in the oncology clinic within a week. Her performance status (PS) was 1 because of her bone pain. She denied any respiratory symptoms. She was a hardly ever smoker but had been a passive smoker due to her son's 20 pack-year smoking history. He was receiving treatment for paranoid schizophrenia. A staging CT scan of the thorax, abdomen and pelvis revealed a left lung primary with hilar node involvement. Histological analysis confirmed an adenocarcinoma, thyroid transcription factor 1 (TTF-1)-positive, *EGFR* wild-type and anaplastic lymphoma kinase (ALK)-negative, consistent with metastatic lung cancer. Her final staging was T4N1M1b. She presented to the emergency department with fever and new left chest pain, 10 days after her bronchoscopy. Her white blood cell count was elevated at $22\times10^9/l$ and her C-reactive protein (CRP) was 3238 nmol/l. A chest X-ray revealed increasing left pleural effusion and patchy consolidation. A CT scan demonstrated a left-sided empyema. A pleural aspirate cultured *Klebsiella pneumoniae* sensitive to co-amoxiclav. A 6 week course of intravenous antibiotics was recommended. After a 2 week inpatient stay she was discharged, with a peripherally inserted central catheter *in situ*, to the care of the virtual ward and community palliative care team to complete her antibiotics and manage her symptom control.

What were the goals of cancer treatment for this patient?

What could be done to reduce the risk of a skeletal–related event?

What is the evidence base for her treatment options?

What other factors might influence her decision to accept active treatment?

What were the goals of cancer treatment for this patient?

The goals of treatment for this woman with metastatic lung cancer with bone involvement were to balance improvement in survival with gains in quality of life (QOL), symptom control and ability to remain at home with her son who had significant mental illness. Her personal goals and values should be sought to assist in joint decision making with regard to treatment, including any desire to undergo treatment as part of a clinical trial.

What could be done to reduce the risk of a skeletal-related event?

Most cases of lung cancer present with advanced disease at diagnosis. Bone metastases are the most frequent secondary site.[1] The presence of synchronous bone metastases from a lung primary reduces prognosis to about 6 months. The risk of a complication is high and its emergence can reduce prognosis and PS further by resulting in increased morbidity, thus precluding any active treatment. The term skeletal-related event refers to five major objective complications of bone cancer disease: the need for radiotherapy to bone, the need for surgery to bone, pathological fracture, metastatic spinal cord compression and hypercalcaemia.[2] Use of a bone-targeted agent such as denosumab or bisphosphonates has become an established method of treating metastatic bone disease. Multiple randomized controlled trials have shown that both these classes of agent effectively reduce skeletal morbidity.[2]

What is the evidence base for her treatment options?

Multiple randomized controlled trials and meta-analyses have established systemic chemotherapy with a doublet combination with a platinum agent for patients with advanced non-small-cell lung carcinoma (NSCLC) and a good PS of 0 or 1, as first line treatment in terms of improving overall survival and symptom control.[3] In these studies the underlying histological subtype did not influence the choice of agent with platinum; instead, clinicians chose the second agent based on the toxicity profile.[4,5] In 2008, a randomized controlled trial with a preplanned analysis for efficacy of histology with chemotherapy agent demonstrated superior overall survival for patients whose cancers had non-squamous histopathology treated with pemetrexed plus cisplatin compared with those with a squamous histopathology treated with gemcitabine plus cisplatin.[6] Four cycles of cisplatin or carboplatin combined with pemetrexed would therefore be the treatment of choice in this case.

In 2010, a novel randomized controlled trial demonstrated that patients with newly diagnosed advanced NSCLC who were randomized to receive early palliative care had significant improvements in both QOL and mood.[7] A striking and unsuspected finding was that although fewer patients in the early palliative care group, compared with the standard care group, received aggressive systemic anticancer chemotherapy, median survival was longer in the early palliative care group. There is emerging evidence that the use of denosumab alone without systemic chemotherapy may improve survival in patients with lung cancer and bone metastases.[8] The question of whether denosumab added to upfront systemic chemotherapy may impact on survival is now the subject of an international randomized controlled trial called Survival Improvement in Lung Cancer Induced by Denosumab Therapy (SPLENDOUR), sponsored by the European Organisation for Research and Treatment of Cancer.[9]

In 2002, Schiller et al.[5] randomly allocated 1207 chemotherapy-naive patients with advanced lung cancer to one of four doublet regimens: cisplatin plus paclitaxel, cisplatin plus gemcitabine, cisplatin plus docetaxel, or carboplatin plus paclitaxel. The 19% response rate was similar across all four regimens, with median survival of 7.9 months. Survival at 1 year was 33% and at 2 years 11%. None of the four regimens offered a significant advantage over the others.[5]

In 2008, Scagliotti *et al.*[6] randomly allocated 1725 chemotherapy-naive patients with stage IIIB or stage IV NSCLC to receive cisplatin plus pemetrexed or cisplatin plus gemcitabine, with a preplanned analysis after stratification for histological subtype. Overall survival was statistically superior for cisplatin plus pemetrexed vs cisplatin plus gemcitabine ($n=847$; 12.6 vs 10.9 months). Overall survival was superior in patients with squamous cell histology ($n=473$; 10.8 vs 9.4 months).

In 2010, Temel *et al.*[7] randomly assigned 151 newly diagnosed patients with metastatic NSCLC to receive early palliative care integrated into standard oncology care, or standard oncology care alone. The primary outcome was change in QOL at 12 weeks. Twenty-seven patients had died by 12 weeks. Of the remaining patients assessed (86%), those assigned to early palliative care had higher scores on the Functional Assessment of Cancer Therapy–Lung scale, indicating better QOL (98.0 vs 91.5, $p=0.03$). Fewer patients in the early palliative care group had depressive symptoms (16% vs 38%, $p=0.05$), and median survival was longer in this group (11.6 vs 8.9 months, $p=0.02$).

What other factors might influence her decision to accept active treatment?

The presence of active infection in this patient requiring intravenous antibiotics prohibited the safe administration of systemic treatment. This is due to the risks of myelosuppression associated with the therapy, which may delay recovery from the infection. Concurrent comorbidity can impact on overall PS. A population-based study in patients with lung cancer who were ≥24 years old and who had started their first cycle of systemic anticancer therapy (SACT) showed the 30 day mortality rate was higher for patients with PS 2–4 compared with those with PS 0.[10]

The care and welfare of her son was at the forefront of our patient's mind, as she feared that any further prolonged inpatient stays would potentially precipitate his admission to a psychiatric unit. In this case the patient was able to articulate precisely what mattered to her most when facing treatment choices for an incurable disease.[11]

After correction of a low vitamin D level she started denosumab, a fully human anti-receptor activator of nuclear factor kappa-B ligand (RANKL) monoclonal antibody, as a monthly subcutaneous injection. The resulting resolution of her painful bone metastases meant her desire for active treatment outside the context of a clinical trial waned. If this had not been as effective, her decisions about other treatment might have altered.

She had read about the development of immunotherapy as a treatment for lung cancer and wanted to recover from this episode to have an opportunity to have her eligibility considered for a clinical trial. The community and virtual ward teams enabled her to be cared for at home so that she could remain with her son.

Conclusion and learning points

- For patients with a good PS, immunohistological confirmation with specific mutational testing of the tumour biopsy is essential for guiding optimum treatment.

- For patients with *EGFR* wild-type and ALK-negative tumours, a doublet combination of a platinum plus pemetrexed is the standard of care for patients with an adenocarcinoma or non-squamous histology, and platinum plus gemcitabine for those with squamous cell cancers.

- Bone metastases are a common site of secondary cancer in patients with lung cancer and their presence can negatively affect prognosis. Targeting bone metastases with a bone-targeted agent can significantly reduce the risk of skeletal-related events.

- Median survival in patients with NSCLC has improved significantly over the last decade, yet remains a deadly disease; therefore, a focus on active symptom control is imperative to ensure optimum QOL.

- Early palliative care integrated into SACT in patients with advanced NSCLC improves QOL and survival.

- Combination chemotherapy has superior outcomes and should be considered first line.

References

1   Katakami N, Kunikane H, Takeda K, *et al.* Prospective study on the incidence of bone metastasis (BM) and skeletal-related events (SREs) in patients (pts) with stage IIIB and IV lung cancer-CSP-HOR 13. *J Thorac Oncol* 2014; 9: 231–8.

2   Coleman R, Body J, Aapro M, *et al.* Bone health in cancer patients: ESMO clinical practice guidelines. *Ann Oncol* 2014; 25 (suppl 3): iii124–37.

3   Coleman RE, McCloskey EV. Bisphosphonates in oncology. *Bone* 2011; 49: 71.

4   NSCLC Meta-Analyses Collaborative Group. Chemotherapy in addition to supportive care improves survival in advanced non-small-cell lung cancer: a systematic review and meta-analysis of individual patient data from 16 randomized controlled trials. *J Clin Oncol* 2008; 26: 4617–25.

5   Schiller J, Harrington D, Belani C, *et al.* Comparison of four chemotherapy regimens for advanced non–small-cell lung cancer. *N Engl J Med* 2002; 346: 92–8.

6   Scagliotti GV, Parikh P, von Pawel J, *et al.* Phase III study comparing cisplatin plus gemcitabine with cisplatin plus pemetrexed in chemotherapy-naive patients with advanced-stage non-small-cell lung cancer. *J Clin Oncol* 2008; 26: 3543–51.

7   Temel JS, Greer JA, Muzikansky A, *et al.* Early palliative care for patients with metastatic non-small-cell lung cancer. *N Engl J Med* 2010; 363: 733–42.

8   Udagawa H, Niho S, Kirita K, *et al.* Impact of denosumab use on the survival of untreated non-squamous non-small cell lung cancer patients with bone metastases. *J Cancer Res Clin Oncol* 2017; 143: 1475–82.

9   European Organisation for Research and Treatment of Cancer. *ETOP/EORTC trial to evaluate denosumab for treating patients with non-small cell lung cancer.* Available from: www.eortc.org/news/etopeortc-trial-to-evaluate-denosumab-for-treating-patients-with-advanced-non-small-cell-lung-cancer (accessed 16 February 2017).

10 Wallington M, Saxon E, Dodwell D. 30-day mortality after systemic anticancer chemotherapy for breast and lung cancer in England: a population-based, observational study. *Lancet Oncol* 2016; 17: 1203–16.

11 Puts MT, Tapscott B, Fitch M, *et al.* A systematic review of factors influencing older adults' decision to accept or decline cancer treatment. *Cancer Treat Rev* 2015; 41: 197–215.

Further reading

- Foglino S, Bravi F, Carretta E, *et al.* The relationship between integrated care and cancer patient experience: a scoping review of the evidence. *Health Policy* 2016; 120: 55–63.

- National Institute for Health and Care Excellence (2011). *Lung cancer: diagnosis and management. Clinical guideline CG121.* Available from: www.nice.org.uk/guidance/cg121 (accessed 30 January 2017).

- National Institute for Health and Care Excellence (2012). *Denosumab for the prevention of skeletal-related events in adults with bone metastases from solid tumours. Technology appraisal guidance TA265.* Available from: www.nice.org.uk/guidance/ta265 (accessed 30 January 2017).

11 Management of Psychological and Behavioural Challenges in a Patient with Glioblastoma

Suryanarayana Kakkilaya, Jane Younger

Case history

A 41-year-old man with stage IV glioblastoma on corticosteroid treatment presented with bizarre behaviour. He was laughing incongruously and screaming at moving traffic outside his house. He also threatened a member of the public. His wife contacted his clinical nurse specialist. An urgent psychiatric review was arranged and the patient was reviewed on the same day by a senior trainee psychiatrist in the psychological medicine department.

The dosage of dexamethasone had been increased from 4 mg to 6 mg per day 1 week earlier. The patient had observed relief from headache but the change in his behaviour started shortly after. There was nothing significant in his medical and psychiatric history. On examination the patient was found to have psychomotor agitation, pressure of speech, lability of mood and paranoid delusions. A diagnosis of organic mood disorder was made with steroids as a contributing factor. A risk assessment identified a risk of further deterioration of his mental health and a high risk of impulsive behaviour. There was a potential risk to others including his two children who lived at home with him. The treatment plan included plans to minimize these risks.

Following consultation with the oncologist, the psychological medicine team decided to reduce the dose of steroid by half and prescribed quetiapine (an antipsychotic medication used in the treatment of manic episode) and zopiclone (a sleeping tablet). The patient gradually improved over a period of 2 weeks, after which he was advised to stop taking the sleeping tablet and to continue with the quetiapine.

What were the challenges in the management of this patient?

How were the risks in the community managed?

What is the evidence base for the treatment of steroid-induced mania?

What are the contributing factors for the development of psychiatric disorder?

What were the challenges in the management of this patient?

There were number of challenges in the management of this patient.

Psychiatric emergency

Manic episodes typically develop suddenly and result in behavioural disturbance often raising concerns for others' safety. Patients suffering from a first episode of acute mania are likely to get arrested for breach of the peace or detained under section 136 of the Mental Health Act (powers given to police to transport an individual to a place of safety for a mental health assessment). This can be very distressing to patients and their family. In this case, due to the timely response from the clinical nurse specialist and the psychological medicine team, police involvement was avoided.

Supporting the family
During a manic episode, it can be difficult to communicate with a patient due to elated mood and poor engagement. This can be a frightening experience for family members. The Maggie's Centre, which is on the site of Clatterbridge Cancer Centre, offered support and information to family members.

Working with the multidisciplinary team
The patient needed close monitoring of both his physical and mental health. The psychological medicine department, the mental health home treatment team, the clinical nurse specialist, the oncologist and the Maggie's Centre were all involved in his care.

How were the risks in the community managed?
Risk assessment is part of mental health assessment. All patients under the care of secondary mental health services will have a care plan that includes a risk assessment and risk management plan. A brief summary of a risk assessment and risk management plan is shown in Table 11.1.

Table 11.1 Summary of the risk assessment and risk management plan.

Domains of risk	Identified risk	Risk management plan
Risk to health	Not sleeping and distressed, which can lead to poor prognosis if not treated early	Pharmacological treatment to help with elated mood and insomnia
		Mental health home treatment team can visit him daily to monitor compliance and side effects
Risk to self	Vulnerability due to inappropriate behaviour He is prone to accidents	His wife and father agreed to be with him and contact emergency services if needed
		Home treatment team practitioner will liaise with the family on a regular basis to monitor risks
Risk to others	High risk of impulsive behaviour, loud and can appear intimidating to others Children may feel scared Also potential risk of accidental harm to others	His family members have agreed to be with him all the time and monitor him closely
		Family members were made aware of the potential risk to children and they agreed to provide extra support
		Home treatment team practitioner will liaise with family on a regular basis to monitor risks

What is the evidence base for the treatment of steroid–induced mania?

Consideration should be given to reduce and stop the steroid.[1] This can be difficult in some patients as it may worsen the physical symptoms. Case reports have shown a good response to haloperidol, risperidone, quetiapine, olanzapine, lithium, lamotrigine, sodium valproate and clonazepam. In some cases, a combination of antipsychotic medication and benzodiazepine may be required.[2] The antipsychotic or mood-stabilizing medication may have to be continued through the course of steroid treatment or as a preventative measure before steroids are prescribed.[3]

What are the contributing factors for the development of psychiatric disorder?

Brain tumours can cause personality change[4] but rarely cause mania.[5] Right frontal lobe tumours are associated with mania, and left frontal lobe lesions are associated with depression.[6] Several studies have shown a direct link between corticosteroids and mania. There is a temporal relation between the starting of steroids and the onset of psychiatric disorder. One study showed a median time of onset of 11.5 days.[1] The psychiatric effects seem to be dose-dependent.[7] The incidence of major psychiatric symptoms in cancer patients treated with high-dose corticosteroids was found to be between 5% and 10%.[8] One review, however, found the incidence of some degree of manic episode to be as high as 35% in patients taking corticosteroids.[9] Surprisingly, a history of psychiatric disorder does not increase the risk of developing a psychiatric adverse reaction to steroid treatment.[8]

Conclusion and learning points

- Consider prescribing a prophylactic mood stabilizer (lithium) before prescribing high-dose steroids in patients with a history of psychosis.

- Inform the patient and family member(s) about potential side effects and whom to contact if necessary.

- Good communication between the different teams involved in the patient's care is essential for delivering patient-centred, integrated care.

- Antipsychotic medication or mood stabilizers are effective in controlling the symptoms of steroid-induced mania. A benzodiazepine may also be required for immediate control of symptoms.

References

1 Lewis DA, Smith RE. Steroid-induced psychiatric syndromes. A report of 14 cases and a review of the literature. *J Affect Disord* 1983; 5: 319–32.

2 Kenna HA, Poon AW, de los Angeles CP, Koran LM. Psychiatric complications of treatment with corticosteroids: review with case report. *Psychiatry Clin Neurosci* 2011; 65: 549–60.

3 Falk WE, Mahnke MW, Poskanzer DC. Lithium prophylaxis of corticotropin-induced psychosis. *JAMA* 1979; 241: 1011–12.

4 Chambers SK, Grassi L, Hyde MK, *et al.* Integrating psychosocial care into neuro-oncology: challenges and strategies. *Front Oncol* 2015; 5: 41.

5 Starkstein SE, Mayberg HS, Berthier ML, *et al.* Mania after brain injury: neuroradiological and metabolic findings. *Ann Neurol* 1990; 27: 652–9.

6 Belyi BI. Mental impairment in unilateral frontal tumours: role of the laterality of the lesion. *Int J Neurosci* 1987; 32: 799–810.

7 Chan L, French ME, Oliver DO, Morris PJ. High- and low-dose prednisolone. *Transplant Proc* 1981; 13: 336–8.

8 Stiefel FC, Breitbart WS, Holland JC. Corticosteroids in cancer: neuropsychiatric complications. *Cancer Invest* 1989; 7: 479–91.

9 Sirois F. Steroid psychosis: a review. *Gen Hosp Psychiatry* 2003; 25: 27–33.

12 Psychological Therapy to Aid Tablet Taking in Cancer Treatment

Lesley Seddon, Fiona James, Ruth E. Board

Case history

A 19-year-old woman presented with a cough and was found to have a large mediastinal mass. Investigations confirmed Hodgkin's lymphoma (nodular sclerosing type, stage II disease). She was treated with hybrid chemotherapy and mediastinal radiotherapy, leading to disease remission. She re-presented 7 years later with a palpable cervical lymph node. Further investigation identified widespread relapse of her lymphoma. Holistic needs assessment (HNA) revealed distress and psychological concerns around swallowing. She was treated with four cycles of gemcitabine, dacarbazine, cyclophosphamide, vincristine and prednisolone chemotherapy but her disease progressed. Further lines of chemotherapy including vinblastine, basiliximab, and etoposide, methylprednisolone, cytarabine and cisplatin preceded an allogenic stem cell transplant from her sister. Treatment was complicated by numerous side effects including peripheral neuropathy, premature ovarian failure and osteopenia. She also developed graft versus host disease of the mouth and skin.

Since her relapse she complained of difficulties swallowing tablets and expressed concerns and fears about tablet taking. No organic basis for her dysphagia was found and she was referred to psycho-oncology for assessment and management of symptoms. Assessment confirmed anxiety and dysfunctional thinking about swallowing tablets. She believed she would choke and become ill. The perceived risk of asphyxiation far outweighed the consequences of non-compliance; consequently, adherence to medication had become problematic and patchy. She was struggling with adjustment and the psychological consequences of having recurrent disease and a challenging prognosis. She felt out of control and overwhelmed by two interconnected threats to her very survival and was feeling increasingly helpless. Following a course of cognitive behavioural therapy (CBT) her symptoms improved and swallowing of her supportive medications became manageable. As her disease has progressed she has accessed intermittent support from the psycho-oncology team.

What psychological therapy options were considered in this case?

What is CBT and how did it work in this case?

What are potential barriers to effective therapy?

What is the evidence base for CBT?

How can psychological issues be identified and managed?

What psychological therapy options were considered in this case?

The primary goal was to improve adherence to her essential oral oncology treatment by overcoming difficulties swallowing tablets. Several forms of psychological therapy have demonstrable efficacy in oncology including mindfulness, acceptance and commitment therapy, solution-focused therapy, supportive counselling and CBT. Her adjustment was compromised by dysfunctional thinking and a powerful belief that she could not take tablets. Patient preference for CBT became evident. Collaborative decision making led to agreement on CBT, as it could target her dysfunctional thinking, imagery, anxious preoccupation, and safety behaviours which were maintaining the problematic tablet taking (Figure 12.1). She was well informed and aware of her options having previously attempted self-help.

What is CBT and how did it work in this case?

CBT is a collaborative process between therapist and client during which strengths and vulnerabilities are acknowledged and problems are noticed, elucidated and challenged. It is useful in oncology as it facilitates convergence between intellectual and emotional adjustment.[1-3] Therapy focuses on the present and the factors that maintain a problem rather than on any historical aetiology. CBT helps find person-centred solutions to enduring problems in integrated cancer care by using idiosyncratic maintenance formulation and specific goal setting. CBT is educative: it uses psycho-education to help patients understand what is happening to them; it also emphasizes the importance of experiential learning about the advantages and disadvantages of pertinent thoughts, feelings and behaviours. Guided discovery and dialogue facilitates insight, building on what patients already know, including information they would rather not acknowledge or think about. Behavioural experiments encourage the individual to explore new behaviours, responses and

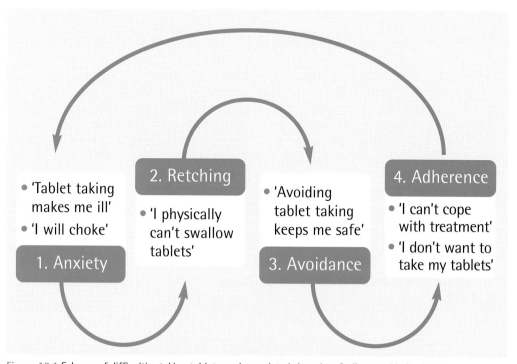

Figure 12.1 Scheme of difficulties taking tablets, and associated thoughts, feelings and behaviours.

alternative ways of thinking. For example, this young woman experimented with dropping her safety behaviours such as avoidance, hanging over the sink or tilting her head back in an exaggerated manner while swallowing. Safety behaviours merely give the illusion of safety, as they only provide temporary relief and the anxiety always recurs. Furthermore, safety behaviours are considered unhelpful because their adoption inhibits experiential learning such as finding that the 'bad thing' did not happen. For example, her belief that she was going to choke remained unchallenged. Thus, the over-reliance on safety behaviours becomes habitual and a dominant feature of a problem maintenance cycle (Figure 12.2).

Challenging unhelpful thinking was an important feature of therapy. The patient was encouraged to notice and identify unhelpful thinking and to respond to it differently. This did not mean positive thinking whereby everything is viewed through rose-tinted glasses but rather she learned to think differently and this had an impact on her affect, mood and cognition. She identified her most upsetting thought and confirmed how much she believed it on a scale of 0–100%. It was established how that made her feel and how strong her emotion was. For example, she had a negative automatic thought, belief or image that she would asphyxiate while taking her medication and she was 90% certain it would happen. She would panic about tablet taking and rated her anxiety level as 90% on a scale of 0–100% (Figure 12.2). This is important, as both the content and belief were rated as high. Another patient may have the same thought but not believe it would

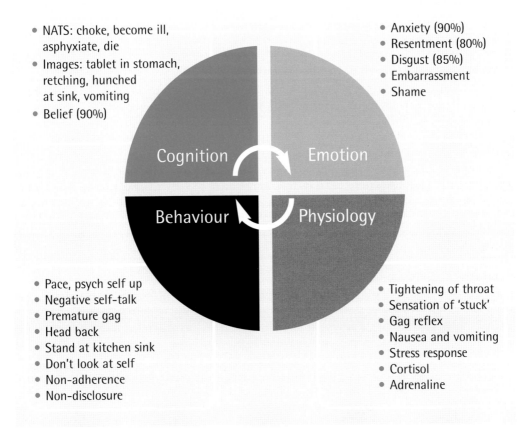

- NATS: choke, become ill, asphyxiate, die
- Images: tablet in stomach, retching, hunched at sink, vomiting
- Belief (90%)

- Anxiety (90%)
- Resentment (80%)
- Disgust (85%)
- Embarrassment
- Shame

Cognition Emotion

Behaviour Physiology

- Pace, psych self up
- Negative self-talk
- Premature gag
- Head back
- Stand at kitchen sink
- Don't look at self
- Non-adherence
- Non-disclosure

- Tightening of throat
- Sensation of 'stuck'
- Gag reflex
- Nausea and vomiting
- Stress response
- Cortisol
- Adrenaline

Figure 12.2 Maintenance formulation of difficulties taking tablets. NAT, negative automatic thought.

happen and therefore may not be anxious about it.

Therapy explored both the belief and content of her distressing thoughts and encouraged the consideration of facts rather than assumptions or beliefs. She compared her mental image of 'swallowing' with an illustration of the anatomical facts. Learning about the physiological swallow guided her to discover that what she thought happened during swallowing was very different from the reality. Having considered the anatomy and physiology of the throat she created an alternative, more helpful image of tablet taking. This challenged her belief that she would asphyxiate and it impacted on her anxiety level. Both were reduced as she checked out the facts, tested the evidence and learned to create constructive, alternative responses to her thoughts. She was also asked to change her safety behaviours and notice what happened. Rather than delaying or standing at the sink retching and coughing she experimented with sitting at the table, as she would at meal times, maintaining a normal head position while swallowing. She learned to observe what happened and how she felt.

Other standard features of CBT were also employed including the use of a contract detailing the session number and duration, venue, record keeping, multidisciplinary liaison, and case supervision. Each session was agenda-led and referred to the case formulation. To ensure continuity over the course of her therapy, sessions were linked with bridging activities including homework.

During therapy the patient's distressing images associated with choking receded significantly. Improvements in the overactivation of her gag reflex and vomiting response were also observed. She achieved a clinically significant reduction in anxious preoccupation associated with problematic tablet taking and was able to adhere to her medical regimen as prescribed.

What are potential barriers to effective therapy?

Heightened anxiety, perceived helplessness and negative affect are problematic and can hinder effective engagement in cancer care. As with any psychological therapy, CBT is not always appropriate and suitability varies considerably.[4] The individual must be psychologically minded and demonstrate an ability to identify with a cognitive model of explanation, along with being receptive to challenge and open to new learning.

Coping with cancer and treatment is a demanding and dynamic process which requires many personal resources. It takes time and is further complicated by recurrence or disease progression. Indeed, if the process of adjustment is ongoing then formal CBT may be inappropriate.[2] Delineating and differentiating normal responses from cancer-related psychological morbidity is complicated and it is important that distress which is proportionate to circumstances be recognized and validated as part of the adjustment process. It helps to normalize rather than pathologize.

What is the evidence base for CBT?

There is considerable support for the effectiveness and benefits of CBT across a range of disorders and populations, giving weight to the empirical status of this form of therapy.[5]

NICE states that prompt assessment of emotional function and referral can minimize the likelihood of cancer-related psychological morbidity and advocates the use of CBT as an appropriate intervention in supportive and palliative care.[6] Meta-analysis data demonstrating the effectiveness of CBT in improving quality of life and reducing psychological morbidity have also been reported, and brief CBT can minimize the risk of depression and anxiety.[3,7] In addition, CBT has been shown to be useful in ameliorating cancer-related pain and distress.[8] Fatigue, sleep disturbance and physical indolence have also responded positively to CBT across the cancer experience, as have illness behaviours and other symptom-related difficulties.[9,10]

In terms of treatment adherence, oral medication is now used more frequently to treat a number of malignancies and side effects. While this has some advantages, oncology treatment can also be compromised by poor compliance.[11] CBT has been shown to be effective in supporting patients in the self-management of their medication.[12] Various approaches have been shown to bolster adherence, including improving behaviours, motivational interviewing and education. Providing interventions that combine these techniques may improve symptom management and medication adherence.[13] This case drew upon the key elements and incorporated them into the person-centred treatment formulation.

How can psychological issues be identified and managed?

It is recommended that psychological issues are reviewed and screened at key points throughout the cancer experience using an HNA. Key screening points include at diagnosis, end of treatment, disease recurrence and any other critical incidents.[1] Psychological screening and review should be an ongoing feature of person-centred, integrated cancer care.[1]

Conclusion and learning points

- Difficulties in taking tablets and poor adherence need to be considered as part of the HNA.

- Distressed patients' adherence to oral treatment needs to be monitored and supported.

- CBT is an effective, evidence-based intervention in cancer care. Mindfulness, solution-focused therapy, supportive counselling, and acceptance and commitment therapy are helpful alternatives.

- Patients who can understand the therapeutic rationale and processes tend to respond better.

- Therapy can be challenging and requires the individual to take risks in terms of facing perceived threats. This involves reducing the reliance on safety behaviours and their illusory benefits.

- Understanding the complex relationship between cognitions, emotions, physiology, behaviours and situational variables is fundamental. It is a precursor to learning and the development of more helpful alternative responses.

References

1 National Institute for Health and Care Excellence. *Guidance on cancer services: improving supportive care for adults with cancer.* London: NICE, 2004.

2 Moorey S, Greer S. *Cognitive behaviour therapy for people with cancer.* Oxford: Oxford University Press, 2002.

3 Osborn R, Demoncada A, Feuerstein M. Psychosocial interventions for depression, anxiety, and quality of life in cancer survivors: meta-analyses. *Int J Psychiatry Med* 2006; 36: 13–34.

4 Safran JD, Segal ZM. *Interpersonal process in cognitive therapy.* New York: Basic Books, 1990.

5 Butler AC, Chapman JE, Forman EM, Beck AT. The empirical status of cognitive-behavioral therapy: a review of meta-analyses. *Clin Psychol Rev* 2006; 26: 17–31.

6 National Institute for Health and Care Excellence. *Early and locally advanced breast cancer: diagnosis and treatment. Clinical guideline CG134.* London: NICE, 2009.

7 Pitceathly C, Maguire P, Fletcher I, *et al.* Can a brief psychological intervention prevent anxiety or depressive disorders in cancer patients? A randomized controlled trial. *Ann Oncol* 2008; 20: 928–34.

8 Tatrow K, Montgomery GH. Cognitive behavioral therapy techniques for distress and pain in breast cancer patients: a meta-analysis. *J Behav Med* 2006; 29: 17–27.

9 Gielissen MF, Verhagen S, Witjes F, Bleijenberg G. Effects of cognitive behavior therapy in severely fatigued disease-free cancer patients compared with patients waiting for cognitive behavior therapy: a randomized controlled trial. *J Clin Oncol* 2006; 24: 4882–7.

10 Given CW, Given B, Champion VL, *et al. Evidence-based behavioral interventions in oncology: state of the knowledge across the cancer care continuum.* New York: Springer, 2003.

11 Bassan F, Peter R, Houbre B, *et al.* Adherence to oral antineoplastic agents by cancer patients: definition and literature review. *Eur J Cancer Care* 2014; 23: 22–35.

12 Ruppar TM, Conn VS, Russell CL. Medication adherence interventions for older adults: literature review. *Res Theory Nurs Pract* 2008; 22: 114–47.

13 Spoelstra S, Burhenn P, DeKoekkoek T, Schueller M. A trial examining an advanced practice nurse intervention to promote medication adherence and symptom management in adult cancer patients prescribed oral anti-cancer agents: study protocol. *J Adv Nurs* 2016; 72: 409–20.

Further reading

- Feros DL, Lane L, Ciarrochi J, Blackledge JT. Acceptance and commitment therapy (ACT) for improving the lives of cancer patients: a preliminary study. *Psychooncology* 2013; 22: 459–64.

- Hulbert-Williams NJ, Storey L, Wilson KG. Psychological interventions for patients with cancer: psychological flexibility and the potential utility of acceptance and commitment therapy. *Eur J Cancer Care* 2015; 24: 15–27.

- Layard R, Clark DM. *Thrive: the power of psychological therapy.* London: Penguin, 2015.

- Mental Health Network, NHS Confederation (2012). *Investing in emotional and psychological wellbeing for patients with long-term conditions.* Available from: www.nhsconfed.org/resources/2012/04/investing-in-emotional-and-psychological-wellbeing-for-patients-with-long-term-conditions (accessed 2 July 2017).

- Wells A. *Cognitive therapy of anxiety disorders: a practice manual and conceptual guide.* Chichester: Wiley, 1995.

- Zhang MF, Wen YS, Liu WY, *et al.* Effectiveness of mindfulness-based therapy for reducing anxiety and depression in patients with cancer: a meta-analysis. *Medicine* 2015; 94: 1–9.

13 Treatment Challenges in a Patient with Metastatic Breast Cancer

Helen Adderley, Elena Takeuchi

Case history

A 54-year-old woman presented with a history of anorexia and fatigue. Seven years previously, she had had a diagnosis of right breast invasive ductal carcinoma, T2 (35 mm), grade 3, N1 (1/11), oestrogen receptor (ER) 75%, progesterone receptor (PR) 24%. Human epidermal growth factor receptor 2 (HER2) was not assayed at that time. She had undergone a right mastectomy and axillary node clearance, followed by adjuvant chemotherapy with epirubicin, cyclophosphamide, methotrexate and fluorouracil, and adjuvant endocrine therapy with tamoxifen. A restaging CT scan confirmed liver metastasis and chest wall recurrence. Biopsy of the chest wall lesion confirmed invasive ductal carcinoma grade 2, ER 7, PR 0, HER2 2+, fluorescence *in situ* hybridization (FISH)-negative. Her liver function test showed mild transaminitis. She was still on tamoxifen at the time of relapse. The patient was well with performance status (PS) 1. Discussions took place about the palliative nature of any treatment that might be considered. Options for available therapy were discussed and she commenced first line palliative chemotherapy with capecitabine.

She was seen by the secondary breast care nurse in clinic, where psychosocial concerns were discussed in detail. This highlighted her anxiety over her husband's mental health and coping mechanisms, as well as her desire to continue to work and maintain 'normality' for as long as possible. She declined community palliative care team support, but regular telephone follow-up by the nurse was offered to identify any additional supportive care needs as she progressed through her treatment course.

A restaging scan after 3 months showed a partial response and she was tolerating capecitabine well. She underwent regular CT and clinical surveillance. Four months later, she developed deranged liver function tests. A restaging CT scan and MRI of the liver confirmed diffuse infiltration of disease in her liver, with new ascites. She became jaundiced and her PS declined rapidly. Discussions took place around what active treatment may be possible in the context of severe liver dysfunction and the patient's wishes and preferred place of care in the event of her continued decline. Reduced-dose weekly paclitaxel was considered and the risks associated with its administration were discussed carefully with the patient. She received one dose but, given her rate of decline, further chemotherapy was ultimately considered futile. She passed away peacefully at home several days later.

What was the aim of treatment in this patient?

What is the evidence base for repeat biopsy in metastatic breast cancer?

What is the evidence for the use of paclitaxel in liver impairment?

What was the role of the supportive care team in this patient's care?

What was the aim of treatment in this patient?

In cases of metastatic breast cancer, patient and clinician goals should be identified to enable joint decision making. The patient's aim was clearly identified: she wished to commence palliative treatment with minimal toxicity, enabling her to maintain 'normality'. At her disease relapse, chemotherapy was chosen over endocrine therapy, as she was already on tamoxifen at the time of disease recurrence and she was symptomatic from her underlying disease and had evidence of liver dysfunction. There was clearly a need to try and get a response quickly. Capecitabine was chosen as an attractive option for first line chemotherapy, due to its favourable side effect profile with little risk of alopecia and less frequent hospital visits. A retrospective study by Kamal et al.[1] demonstrated similar effectiveness of capecitabine versus a taxane when used in metastatic breast cancer. This oral chemotherapy option took the patient's wishes of maintaining 'normality' into consideration.

Despite her initial favourable response to capecitabine, her disease progressed very rapidly and she developed life-threatening hepatic dysfunction. At this point in her disease course, it was clear that her prognosis was very poor; however, given her young age, further chemotherapy was considered with the hope that it might elicit some response. The palliative care team were closely involved to support her through the transition from active therapy to best supportive care.

What is the evidence base for repeat biopsy in metastatic breast cancer?

Identification of HER2 status and hormone receptors, ER and PR, guide treatment planning and inform clinical outcome in both adjuvant and metastatic settings. The role of repeat biopsy to confirm breast cancer metastasis is not mandatory for all cases but has the benefits of excluding benign pathology and other primary malignant disease and evaluating for discordance of biological features. Discordance may result from changes in disease biology, effects of previous treatment, tumour heterogeneity and developments in gene amplification assays. NICE guidance currently recommends assessing hormone receptor and HER2 status at disease recurrence if not assessed at original diagnosis.[2] Repeat biopsy enables targeted, individualized treatment of metastatic disease considering standard of care or clinical trials. When originally diagnosed our patient did not have a HER2 status assay; it was therefore particularly important to evaluate this.

Retrospective analyses have identified discordances between hormone receptor and HER2 status in primary and metastatic breast cancer.[3] A prospective study by Amir et al.,[4] published in 2012, biopsied 121 patients with loco-regional recurrence or distant metastatic disease. An alternative diagnosis including benign disease or second primary was identified in 3.3% of biopsies. Discordance in ER, PR and HER2 status between confirmed primary breast cancer and metastases was 16%, 40% and 10%, respectively. These results have been replicated in the Breast Recurrence in Tissues Study (BRITS), a multicentre prospective study in the UK.[5] Pooled analysis of these studies demonstrated a change in management in 14% of patients after biopsy of metastatic disease.[6]

What is the evidence for the use of paclitaxel in liver impairment?

Patients with advanced disease, liver metastasis and liver dysfunction pose a challenge when deciding suitable chemotherapy regimens. Most clinical trials exclude patients with significant hepatic dysfunction. As paclitaxel is metabolized by the liver and undergoes oxidation by the cytochrome P450 system with biliary clearance,[7] patients with liver dysfunction may be at increased risk of toxicity, particularly grades 3–4 myelosuppression.[8]

The summary of product characteristics recommends reduced dosing in the context of liver dysfunction. Drug companies recommend various dose reductions. The general consensus is that paclitaxel should be avoided if bilirubin is more than five times, or transaminases more than 10 times, the upper limit of normal; the risk–benefit ratio should be reviewed in each individual case.

Our patient was given a dose reduction in an attempt to minimize toxicity, clearly counselled regarding the potential risks, and her liver function tests were closely monitored.

What was the role of the supportive care team in this patient's care?

The supportive care team consisting of secondary breast care nurses and palliative care nurses were involved with our patient's care from the diagnosis of metastatic disease. Early involvement enabled her goals, psychosocial concerns and symptom control needs to be identified in a timely manner. Identifying the patient's treatment aims enabled the physicians and the patient to have open and honest discussions around expectations. Psychological and symptom control support transitioned from secondary breast care nurses to palliative care nurses as her disease progressed. The palliative care nurses supported both the clinicians and the patient, facilitating difficult discussions regarding the uncertainty of second line chemotherapy with no guarantee of response and the transition from active treatment to best supportive care. Although advance care planning was declined until late in the disease trajectory, the supportive care team were able to accommodate the patient's wishes to be cared for at home.

Management of metastatic breast cancer can involve multiple lines of treatment and patients can remain well until a short time before death. Sometimes end-of-life care needs are identified late in the disease course, resulting in a lack of community support and emergency admissions for end-of-life care. In order to address this, The Christie NHS Foundation Trust has developed an integrated medical oncology and palliative breast care team. The team aims to review all patients with metastatic disease and identify holistic aspects of care including: individual needs and concerns of patients, priorities for care, community support, advance care planning, identification of patients in the last year of life, and liaison with other healthcare professionals in the community. Farrell and Coleby[9] demonstrated that during the first 15 months of practice the number of bed days saved in the trust was 1134, and 59 emergency admissions for end-of-life care were avoided.

This integrated approach improved our patient's overall experience and her transition to end-of-life care.

Conclusion and learning points

- In metastatic breast cancer, the aims of both the patient and the physician should be identified to enable open and honest discussion about treatment options, goals of treatment and expectations.

- A biopsy of metastatic disease should be considered at recurrence to enable targeted, individualized treatment to be offered. NICE guidelines advise that biopsy should be performed if initial hormone receptor or HER2 status is unknown.

- Paclitaxel can be used at a reduced dose in metastatic breast cancer patients with liver dysfunction. The summary of product characteristics and local guidelines should be consulted.

- When paclitaxel is used in liver dysfunction, patients should be clearly informed about side effects and the need for close monitoring of liver function tests.
- The supportive care team and palliative breast care team have an important role in supporting patients' psychosocial and physical needs and carrying out advance care planning and holistic needs assessments.

References

1 Kamal AH, Camacho F, Anderson R, *et al*. Similar survival with single-agent capecitabine or taxane in first-line therapy for metastatic breast cancer. *Breast Cancer Res Treat* 2012; 134: 371–8.

2 National Institute for Clinical Excellence (2009). *Advanced breast cancer: diagnosis and treatment. Clinical guideline.* Available from: www.nice.org.uk/guidance/cg81/resources/advanced-breast-cancer-diagnosis-and-treatment-975683850181 (accessed 23 February 2017).

3 Vignot S, Besse B, André F, *et al*. Discrepancies between primary tumour and metastasis: a literature review on clinically established biomarkers. *Crit Rev Oncol Hematol* 2012; 84: 301–13.

4 Amir E, Miller M, Geddie W, *et al*. Prospective study evaluating the impact of tissue confirmation of metastatic disease in patients with breast cancer. *J Clin Oncol* 2012; 30: 587–92.

5 Thompson AM, Jordan LB, Quinlan P, *et al*. Prospective comparison of switches in biomarker status between primary and recurrent breast cancer: the Breast Recurrence in Tissues Study (BRITS). *Breast Cancer Res* 2010; 12: R92.

6 Amir E, Clemons M, Purdie CA, *et al*. Tissue confirmation of disease recurrence in breast cancer patients: pooled analysis of multi-centre, multidisciplinary prospective studies. *Cancer Treat Rev* 2012; 38: 708–14.

7 Cresteil T, Monsarrat B, Alvinerie P, *et al*. Taxol metabolism by human liver microsomes: identification of cytochrome P450 isozymes involved in its biotransformation. *Cancer Res* 1994; 54: 386–92.

8 Wilson WH, Berg SL, Bryant G, *et al*. Paclitaxel in doxorubicin-refractory or mitoxantrone-refractory breast cancer: a phase I/II trial of 96-hour infusion. *J Clin Oncol* 1994; 12: 1621–9.

9 Farrell C, Coleby T. An integrated model for breast cancer and palliative care. *Cancer Nurs Pract* 2016; 15: 28–31.

Further reading

- Carlson RW, Allred DC, Anderson BO, *et al*. Metastatic breast cancer, version 1.2012: featured updates to the NCCN guidelines. *J Natl Compr Canc Netw* 2012; 10: 821–9.

- Criscitiello C, André F, Thompson AM, *et al*. Biopsy confirmation of metastatic sites in breast cancer patients: clinical impact and future perspectives. *Breast Cancer Res* 2014; 16: 205.

- Gold Standards Framework. *Advance care planning.* Available from: www.goldstandardsframework.org.uk/advance-care-planning (accessed 5 February 2017).

- The North London Cancer Network (2009). *Dose adjustments for cytotoxics in hepatic impairment.* Available from: www.londoncancer.org/media/65594/hepatic-impairment-dosage-adjustment-for-cytotoxics.pdf (accessed 5 February 2017).

14 Treatment of Cervical Cancer during Pregnancy and Management of Late Effects

Alexandra Gilbert, Kate Cardale, Galina Velikova

Case history

A 31-year-old woman presented with bleeding at 27 weeks of pregnancy. This was her fourth pregnancy. She had a previously reported abnormal smear (cervical intraepithelial neoplasia), but no further follow-up had been offered. She had no other relevant medical history. On examination she was found to have a visible tumour at the cervix, and a biopsy was taken. Histopathology reported a poorly differentiated squamous cell carcinoma. An MRI scan of the pelvis revealed a 5 cm × 3 cm × 4 cm tumour in the anterior lip of the cervix extending into the left parametrium. A CT scan of the thorax reported no metastatic disease.

The patient had an elective caesarean section in a tertiary care centre at 32 weeks, 5 weeks after diagnosis, and gave birth to a healthy baby. The reassessment MRI and PET-CT scan showed the tumour had grown to 6.0 cm × 6.5 cm, with prolapse into the upper vagina and an abnormal pelvic node: International Federation of Gynecology and Obstetrics (FIGO) stage IIB node-positive squamous cell carcinoma of the cervix.

She was scheduled to have 48 Gy of radiotherapy in 28 fractions and five cycles of weekly concurrent cisplatin chemotherapy, followed by 21 Gy of intracavity brachytherapy in three fractions. It was not, however, possible to deliver the MRI-guided brachytherapy boost to the whole tumour, due to the location of the residual disease. She therefore had an external beam phase 2 boost to the residual tumour volume (18 Gy in 10 fractions and two further, concurrent cisplatin cycles). The potential increase in significant long-term toxicity was discussed with her.

She had a good partial response after 6 weeks of treatment. Routine follow-up at 3 months with post-treatment MRI and a PET-CT scan showed a complete response to treatment, and MRI at 12 months showed no residual or progressive disease.

At baseline, during treatment and in the year following treatment, as part of a clinical study of patient-reported outcomes the patient completed online questionnaires regarding her symptoms and routine clinical care. During treatment she reported expected short-term side effects of fatigue, diarrhoea, urinary frequency and dysuria. These settled but over the next 18 months of follow-up she developed late effects of peripheral neuropathy, urinary incontinence, intermittent haematuria and urgency, bowel urgency and abdominal cramps, hip stiffness and menopausal symptoms. Radiation cystitis was diagnosed following intermittent haematuria symptoms (Figure 14.1). Supportive treatments for those symptoms were given. She has had some benefit from hormone replacement therapy for hot flushes and joint aches; pelvic floor exercises for urinary incontinence; and bowel symptoms are managed with hyoscine butylbromide and loperamide as required. Her peripheral neuropathy symptoms have resolved.

What is the evidence base for postpartum treatment options?

How does the management of cervical cancer differ depending on tumour stage and trimester of pregnancy?

What is the role of PET–CT in staging and response assessment in cervical cancer?

What is the schedule and purpose of routine follow-up after treatment?

How best to identify and manage late effects following pelvic radiotherapy with concurrent chemotherapy

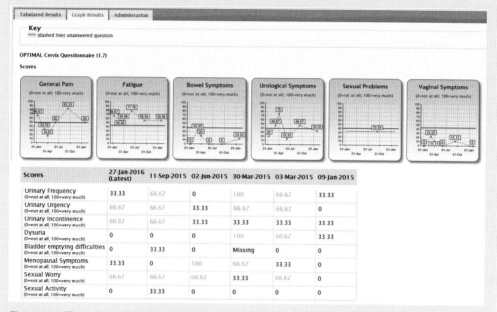

Scores	27-Jan-2016 (Latest)	11-Sep-2015	02-Jun-2015	30-Mar-2015	03-Mar-2015	09-Jan-2015
Urinary Frequency (0=not at all; 100=very much)	33.33	66.67	0	100	66.67	33.33
Urinary Urgency (0=not at all; 100=very much)	66.67	66.67	33.33	66.67	66.67	0
Urinary Incontinence (0=not at all; 100=very much)	66.67	66.67	33.33	33.33	33.33	33.33
Dysuria (0=not at all; 100=very much)	0	0	0	100	66.67	33.33
Bladder emptying difficulties (0=not at all; 100=very much)	0	33.33	0	Missing	0	0
Menopausal Symptoms (0=not at all; 100=very much)	33.33	0	100	66.67	33.33	0
Sexual Worry (0=not at all; 100=very much)	66.67	66.67	66.67	33.33	66.67	0
Sexual Activity (0=not at all; 100=very much)	0	33.33	0	0	0	0

Figure 14.1 Illustrations of the patient's symptoms using European Organisation for Research and Treatment of Cancer (EORTC) QLQ-C30 and EORTC QLQ-CX24 questionnaires. Symptoms are scored 0–100: higher scores correspond to worse symptoms. Combined symptoms presented in the graphs over time with scores above the green line are suggestive of symptoms above a normal threshold. Tabular responses of worse severity are also highlighted in green.

What is the evidence base for postpartum treatment options?

Patients with stage IB2–IV cervical squamous cell carcinoma are offered definitive treatment with external beam radiotherapy and concurrent cisplatin chemotherapy (40 mg/m²), followed by intracavity or interstitial brachytherapy or an external beam boost. A combination of surgery and radiotherapy increases morbidity and should therefore be avoided.[1] Randomized controlled trials have used regimens of 40.0–50.4 Gy in daily 1.8–2.0 Gy fractions.[1,2] A meta-analysis of patients with locally advanced disease found that the addition of platinum-based chemotherapy to radiotherapy alone improved overall survival, as well as local and distant recurrence rates.[3] This was associated with an increase in acute haematological and gastrointestinal toxicity with limited data available on late effects. Overall treatment time, including brachytherapy, should not exceed 56 days for patients with squamous cell carcinoma histology. Haemoglobin levels should be maintained above 120 g/l during treatment to optimize outcomes. Small-volume parametrial disease can be usually be treated with brachytherapy; however, a simultaneous integrated boost may be considered to achieve tumour control, although it is unlikely that three-dimensional conformal radiotherapy would allow normal tissue dose constraints to be met. Recent clinical studies have evaluated the use of image-guided adaptive brachytherapy to improve dose optimization and have found improvements in disease-free survival and local control with associated reductions in toxicity.[4]

How does the management of cervical cancer differ depending on tumour stage and trimester of pregnancy?

Treatment depends on tumour stage and gestational age of the fetus. During pregnancy, radical hysterectomy or pelvic irradiation would result in fetal death and termination of pregnancy; preservation of pregnancy therefore necessarily leads to a modification in management. Close monitoring during the first trimester (weeks 1–12) and up to the end of the second trimester (weeks 13–27) is recommended if the patient wishes to preserve the pregnancy, as systemic treatments are associated with an increased risk of fetal congenital malformations and miscarriage.[5] Chemotherapy given in the second and third trimesters has not been associated with significant fetal defects although an increased risk of fetal and obstetric complications is seen. For patients presenting in the third trimester (weeks 28+), it is recommended that treatment be delayed until after delivery, and early delivery should be considered. This was the approach used in our patient.

In early-stage disease definitive treatment can be deferred until after delivery, providing the patient is closely monitored. For more advanced stages (FIGO stage IB1 and above), radiological staging using pelvic MRI to assess for nodal metastases is used to discriminate between women in whom monitoring is possible and those in whom intermediate treatment is recommended.[6] Clinicians treating node-negative stage IB1 could opt for a period of close monitoring or chemotherapy, followed by surgery after (or, in specialized centres, during) delivery. For locally advanced and high-risk disease, platinum-based chemotherapy followed by definitive treatment after delivery is recommended (cisplatin- or carboplatin-based regimens with or without paclitaxel).[5] Chemotherapy should not be administered after week 33 of pregnancy, to avoid delivery during the nadir period.[6]

What is the role of PET-CT in staging and response assessment in cervical cancer?

PET-CT has been found to improve the sensitivity and specificity of cervical cancer staging, particularly with respect to nodal involvement and distant metastatic disease. There is emerging evidence that the use of PET-CT in metabolic response assessment at 3 months can predict long-term outcomes.[7] PET-CT is already the standard of care for response assessment in the treatment of fluorodeoxyglucose (FDG)-avid lymphoma.

What is the schedule and purpose of routine follow-up after treatment?

Follow-up is aimed at early identification of recurrence, to improve survival and to support the long-term consequences of treatment. Clinical follow-up generally involves consultations every

3 months for the first 2 years, extending to every 6 months, then yearly to complete 5 years of follow-up. Imaging (MRI +/− PET-CT) at 3 months then at 1 year is designed to assess response and detect asymptomatic recurrence. However, the protocols in place to detect recurrence are not evidence-based and there is no evidence that the current model identifies recurrence earlier or impacts survival. Multiple hospital visits may be anxiety generating for patients and the cost-effectiveness is questionable.

In cervical cancer the majority of recurrences are symptomatic. Use of patient-reported outcomes in clinical practice has been proposed as an adjunct/alternative to routine clinical follow-up. Potentially the use of patient-reported outcomes could screen for late adverse events and help detect recurrences, thus supporting individual patient care in a cost-effective way from a healthcare system perspective.[8]

How best to identify and manage late effects following pelvic radiotherapy with concurrent chemotherapy

Currently there is poor recognition of the extent of acute and late adverse events following pelvic radiotherapy, and minimal research to guide optimal management of patients. The commonest late toxicities reported after pelvic radiotherapy for cervical cancer are bowel, urinary and sexual dysfunction along with musculoskeletal adverse events and lymphoedema. These adverse events are highlighted in studies using different methodological approaches ranging from randomized controlled trials to qualitative research, and their impact on patients' quality of life has been well documented.

Evidence that the integration of patient-reported outcomes can improve the accuracy, quality and efficiency of adverse event data collection has led to the recommendations to include patient-reported outcome data collection alongside clinician reporting in cancer clinical trials. Research has found that using patient-reported outcomes in clinical follow-up to measure symptomatic toxicity can improve monitoring of symptoms and enhance communication without extending the duration of the consultation.[9] The patient-reported outcome results can be used to structure the consultations and may act as an ice-breaker to discuss challenging symptoms such as sexual dysfunction. Guidance on how to incorporate patient-reported outcomes in routine clinical practice is now available.[10,11]

Clear guidance on the investigation and management of gastrointestinal symptoms is also available.[12] For patients with bowel frequency, urgency and incontinence, initial clinical management includes discussion about the use of antidiarrhoeal medication, pelvic floor exercises and ensuring fibre intake is not excessive. Appropriate investigations include screening bloods, including vitamin B_{12}, folate, ferritin, thyroid function tests and glucose, and sending a stool sample for culture. Nocturnal bowel opening and toilet dependency warrant referral to a gastroenterologist for further investigation.

Urinary adverse events if troublesome are commonly referred to a urogynaecologist for further investigation. Simple measures such as discussion of pelvic floor exercises can be carried out in the clinic. Sexual dysfunction following pelvic radiotherapy is complex and there is little research into the best management of symptoms.[13] Vaginal stenosis and vaginal dryness are common and are exacerbated by loss of fertility during treatment and an early menopause. There may also, however, be complex psychological issues around resuming sexual activity following treatment. Vaginal dilators are recommended to be used as soon as comfortable after completion of treatment, with the aim of reducing the risk of vaginal stenosis to aid both sexual activity and clinical follow-up. Use of vaginal moisturizers and oestrogen creams as well as hormone replacement therapy can also help lubrication and reduce vaginal dryness. Severe vaginal stenosis may require referral for surgical dilation. Psychosexual concerns can often be supported by a clinical nurse specialist with psychological training, or be referred to a psychosexual counsellor.

Conclusion and learning points

- Treatment with concurrent chemoradiotherapy followed by brachytherapy has superior outcomes and should be considered first line.
- Individualization of treatment may be necessary for patients with extensive tumours requiring phase 2 management with an external beam boost rather than brachytherapy.
- Optimal management of patients diagnosed with cervical cancer during pregnancy requires consideration of gestational age and tumour stage.
- PET-CT improves initial staging of FDG-avid tumours through greater sensitivity and specificity for involved nodes and distant metastases.
- Response assessment PET-CT has an emerging role in the prediction of long-term outcomes in cervical cancer.
- Protocols of clinical follow-up are not evidence-based.
- Patient-reported outcomes collected in routine clinical practice can be used to identify acute and late effects following pelvic radiotherapy, enhance communication between patient and physician, and lead to appropriate management.
- Management of late effects following pelvic radiotherapy is multidisciplinary. More information on the extent of acute and late effects following radiotherapy is required to guide further research on evidence-based interventions.

References

1   Landoni F, Maneo A, Colombo A, et al. Randomised study of radical surgery versus radiotherapy for stage Ib–IIa cervical cancer. Lancet 1997; 350: 535–40.

2   Peters WA 3rd, Liu PY, Barrett RJ 2nd, et al. Concurrent chemotherapy and pelvic radiation therapy compared with pelvic radiation therapy alone as adjuvant therapy after radical surgery in high-risk early-stage cancer of the cervix. J Clin Oncol 2000; 18: 1606–13.

3   Chemoradiotherapy for Cervical Cancer Meta-Analysis Collaboration (CCCMAC). Reducing uncertainties about the effects of chemoradiotherapy for cervical cancer: a systematic review and meta-analysis of individual patient data from 18 randomized trials. J Clin Oncol 2008; 26: 5802–12.

4   Potter R, Georg P, Dimopoulos JC, et al. Clinical outcome of protocol based image (MRI) guided adaptive brachytherapy combined with 3D conformal radiotherapy with or without chemotherapy in patients with locally advanced cervical cancer. Radiother Oncol 2011; 100: 116–23.

5   Fruscio R, Villa A, Chiari S, et al. Delivery delay with neoadjuvant chemotherapy for cervical cancer patients during pregnancy: a series of nine cases and literature review. Gynecol Oncol 2012; 126: 192–7.

6   Peccatori FA, Azim HA Jr, Orecchia R, et al. Cancer, pregnancy and fertility: ESMO clinical practice guidelines for diagnosis, treatment and follow-up. Ann Oncol 2013; 24 (suppl 6): vi160–70.

7 Scarsbrook A, Vaidyanathan S, Chowdhury F, *et al.* Efficacy of qualitative response assessment interpretation criteria at 18F-FDG PET-CT for predicting outcome in locally advanced cervical carcinoma treated with chemoradiotherapy. *Eur J Nucl Med Mol Imaging* 2017; 44: 581–8.

8 Gilbert A, Sebag-Montefiore D, Davidson S, Velikova G. Use of patient-reported outcomes to measure symptoms and health related quality of life in the clinic. *Gynecol Oncol* 2015; 136: 429–39.

9 Velikova G, Booth L, Smith AB, *et al.* Measuring quality of life in routine oncology practice improves communication and patient well-being: a randomized controlled trial. *J Clin Oncol* 2004; 22: 714–24.

10 International Society for Quality of Life Research (2015). *User's guide to implementing patient-reported outcomes assessment in clinical practice.* Available from: www.isoqol.org/UserFiles/2015UsersGuide-Version2.pdf (accessed 1 May 2017).

11 European Organisation for Research and Treatment of Cancer (2016). *EORTC Quality of Life Group: manual for the use of EORTC measures in daily clinical practice.* Available from: http://groups.eortc.be/qol/manuals (accessed 1 May 2017).

12 Andreyev HJ, Davidson SE, Gillespie C, *et al.* Practice guidance on the management of acute and chronic gastrointestinal problems arising as a result of treatment for cancer. *Gut* 2012; 61: 179–92.

13 Denton AS, Maher EJ. Interventions for the physical aspects of sexual dysfunction in women following pelvic radiotherapy. *Cochrane Database Syst Rev* 2003; 1: CD003750.

CASE STUDY

15 A Patient with Prostate Cancer with Ureteric Obstruction and Complex Social Issues

Charlotte Richardson, Iva Damyanova

Case history

A 65-year-old man attended the urology-oncology clinic. He had recently been diagnosed with Gleason 9 (4+5) adenocarcinoma of the prostate with bone metastases and pelvic lymphadenopathy and had been commenced on androgen deprivation therapy (ADT). His presenting prostate-specific antigen (PSA) level was 200 µg/l. He was symptomatic from his spinal metastases, reporting low back pain. He had tried paracetamol with minimal effect.

His comorbidities included type 2 diabetes and hypertension. He also had chronic kidney disease secondary to diabetic nephropathy; his normal baseline creatinine level was 140 µmol/l. A staging CT scan at diagnosis showed evidence of left-sided hydronephrosis secondary to extensive pelvic lymphadenopathy and acute kidney injury.

He was the main carer for his disabled wife and did not have any close family or friends in the area for support. He took her out every day to a small café in his neighbourhood.

The option for upfront chemotherapy with six cycles of docetaxel was discussed in clinic. He initially declined treatment, however, as he was concerned about leaving his wife alone while he was having chemotherapy. He was also worried about the risk of neutropenic sepsis, as if it was necessary to admit him to hospital there was no one else to care for his wife. In view of his concerns and social circumstances we made several modifications which enabled him to go ahead with chemotherapy.

We prescribed prophylactic granulocyte-colony stimulating factor (GCSF) to minimize the risk of febrile neutropenia with the aim to prevent hospital admissions.

We commenced his docetaxel chemotherapy at the recommended dose of 75 mg/m² but monitored him closely for signs of neuropathy which might have impaired his ability to care for his wife.

We organized for his wife to be seen by a social worker and occupational therapist, and to have regular home care visits.

We arranged for hospital transport to take him and his wife to the chemotherapy appointments so he did not have to leave her at home.

The urology multidisciplinary team discussed the management of his ureteric obstruction and decided that he should have a temporary nephrostomy, with the plan to convert to a stent if he had a good response to chemotherapy and ADT.

The patient successfully completed six cycles of docetaxel with no adverse effects. He did not require any hospital admissions during his treatment. A CT scan at the end of treatment showed resolution of his pelvic lymphadenopathy and his PSA fell from 200 to 1.5 µg/l. He successfully underwent a metallic ureteric stent insertion and his renal function returned to baseline.

What was the goal of cancer treatment for this patient?

What is the evidence base for his treatment options?

How did his social issues affect the decision to give chemotherapy?

How do we manage ureteric obstruction in patients with malignancy?

What was the goal of cancer treatment for this patient?

The aim of upfront chemotherapy for this patient was to improve overall survival, delay progression on ADT, delay the need for further treatment, and reduce the likelihood of complications from his disease (especially obstructive uropathy). There is evidence that upfront docetaxel increases the time before patients experience a significant skeletal event by up to 7 months.[1] These potential benefits, however, need to be weighed up against the risk of side effects, particularly the risk of permanent peripheral neuropathy and worsening quality of life (QOL).

What is the evidence base for his treatment options?

Evidence for the use of docetaxel in castrate-resistant prostate cancer (CRPC) is well established. The TAX 327 trial[2] compared docetaxel plus prednisone with mitoxantrone plus prednisone. The results, published in 2004, showed that docetaxel improved overall survival by 2.4 months (16.5 vs 18.9 months) and produced a greater improvement in QOL. Docetaxel is now the standard of care for patients with metastatic CRPC and can be used either before or after novel hormone treatments (abiraterone or enzalutamide).

Three recent trials have investigated using upfront docetaxel rather than waiting until patients develop CRPC.

A UK-based randomized controlled trial, Systemic Therapy in Advancing or Metastatic Prostate Cancer: Evaluation of Drug Efficacy – a Multi-Stage Multi-Arm Randomised Controlled Trial (STAMPEDE),[3] recruited 2962 patients with a new diagnosis of castrate-naive prostate cancer. Patients were randomized 2:1:1:1 to ADT alone vs ADT plus zoledronic acid vs ADT plus docetaxel vs ADT plus docetaxel plus zoledronic acid. The addition of docetaxel compared with ADT alone improved overall survival by 10 months (71 vs 81 months; HR 0.78; 95% CI 0.66, 0.93; $p<0.006$). A subgroup analysis of patients with metastatic disease showed a 15 month improvement in overall survival ($p=0.005$). Therefore, upfront docetaxel appears to be more beneficial in patients with a high burden of disease. Adding zoledronic acid to docetaxel did not add any statistically significant advantage in men with or without metastatic prostate cancer ($p=0.592$).

A US phase III randomized controlled trial, Androgen Ablation Therapy with or without Chemotherapy in Treating Patients with Metastatic Prostate Cancer (CHAARTED),[4] recruited 790 patients with castrate-naive prostate cancer. Patients were randomized to ADT alone vs ADT plus docetaxel. Median overall survival was 13.6 months longer with ADT plus docetaxel (57.6 vs 44.0 months; HR 0.61; 95% CI 0.47, 0.80; $p<0.001$). The time to progression was also increased (20.2

vs 11.7 months; HR 0.61; 95% CI 0.51, 0.72; $p<0.001$). The incidence of grade 3 and 4 toxicities, however, was increased with docetaxel compared with ADT alone; the rate of grade 3–4 febrile neutropenia was 6.2% and the rate of peripheral neuropathy was 0.5%.

A French study, Hormone Therapy and Docetaxel or Hormone Therapy Alone in Treating Patients with Metastatic Prostate Cancer (GETUG-AFU 15),[5] randomized 385 patients with castrate-naive prostate cancer to either ADT alone or ADT plus docetaxel. Contrary to the STAMPEDE and CHAARTED trials, this study showed no survival benefit with docetaxel compared with ADT alone (48.6 vs 48.6 months; HR 0.88; 95% CI 0.68, 1.14; $p=0.3$). A retrospective analysis, however, showed a 14 month improvement in overall survival in patients with a high burden of disease.

How did his social issues affect the decision to give chemotherapy?

In order to give this patient upfront docetaxel, which is now the gold standard treatment, several social issues had to be resolved.

- We arranged a package of care for his wife so that she would not need to rely on her husband as much for help with home care; therefore, if he struggled with chemotherapy side effects he would be able to rest after treatment.

- We organized a review by the occupational therapy team to make any necessary modifications to his home, again to make it easier to care for his wife.

- We arranged hospital transport to bring him and his wife to the chemotherapy department so that he did not need to leave his wife alone while having treatment.

- We arranged for him to have input from the Macmillan community nurses for help with managing his bone pain and providing psychological support.

- We added prophylactic GCSF to his chemotherapy regimen to minimize the risk of neutropenic sepsis and thus try to prevent hospital admissions.

How do we manage ureteric obstruction in patients with malignancy?

Ureteric obstruction is common in patients with cancer. It occurs most frequently in patients with urological or gynaecological cancers; in patients with prostate cancer it is usually due to pelvic lymphadenopathy. It is associated with frequent upper urinary tract infections or renal failure and if untreated could be fatal.

There are several options for managing ureteric obstruction. These include a retrograde ureteric stent, an antegrade ureteric stent, long-term nephrostomy, or deciding not to intervene and taking a best supportive care approach. Antegrade stent insertion is much more likely to be successful compared with retrograde ureteric stent insertion.[6] Retrograde ureteric stent insertion is rarely attempted in patients with prostate cancer due to the high rate of failure. The likelihood of complications occurring is usually the same for both procedures. Long-term nephrostomy is less likely to be acceptable to patients. A trial by Wilson et al.[7] showed that less than half of patients felt they had a good QOL with a long-term nephrostomy. It is therefore important that all decisions about management of ureteric obstruction are discussed in detail with patients, as they may prefer to receive best supportive care rather than undergo intervention.

In our patient's case, it was felt that a temporary nephrostomy prior to his chemotherapy would be appropriate to minimize the risk of upper urinary tract infections and to improve his renal function in the short term. An antegrade ureteric stent was inserted, as he had a good response to chemotherapy.

Conclusion and learning points

- Upfront chemotherapy with six cycles of docetaxel at the time of diagnosis of castrate-naive prostate cancer has been shown to improve overall and progression-free survival and delay complications of disease.

- The management of ureteric obstruction in malignancy is complex and patients need to be fully informed regarding treatment options.

- Social issues need to be carefully considered prior to commencing patients on chemotherapy.

References

1 Medical Research Council, Clinical Trials Unit (2015). *Upfront docetaxel for men with prostate cancer.* Available from: www.ctu.mrc.ac.uk/13706/13710/docetaxel_prostate_cancer (accessed 17 July 2017).

2 Tannock I, de Wit R, Berry W, *et al.* Docetaxel plus prednisone or mitoxantrone plus prednisone for advanced prostate cancer. *N Engl J Med* 2004; 351: 1502–12.

3 James ND, Sydes MR, Clarke NW, *et al.* Addition of docetaxel, zoledronic acid, or both to first-line long-term hormone therapy in prostate cancer (STAMPEDE): survival results from an adaptive, multiarm, multistage, platform randomised controlled trial. *Lancet* 2016; 387: 1163–77.

4 Sweeney CJ, Chen YH, Carducci M, *et al.* Chemohormonal therapy in metastatic hormone-sensitive prostate cancer. *N Engl J Med* 2015; 373: 737–46.

5 Gravis G, Fizazi K, Joly F, *et al.* Androgen-deprivation therapy alone or with docetaxel in non-castrate metastatic prostate cancer (GETUG-AFU 15): a randomised, open-label, phase 3 trial. *Lancet Oncol* 2013; 14: 149–58.

6 Chitale S, Scott-Barrett S, Burgess N. The management of ureteric obstruction secondary to malignant pelvic disease. *Clin Radiol* 2002; 57: 1118–21.

7 Wilson J, Urwin G, Stower M. The role of percutaneous nephrostomy in malignant ureteric obstruction. *Ann R Coll Surg Engl* 2005; 87: 21–4.

Further reading

- European Society for Medical Oncology (2016). *Cancer of the prostate: ESMO clinical practice guidelines.* Available from: www.esmo.org/Guidelines/Genitourinary-Cancers/Cancer-of-the-Prostate (accessed 17 July 2017).

- National Institute for Health and Care Excellence (2016). *Hormone-sensitive metastatic prostate cancer. Evidence summary ESUOM50.* Available from: www.nice.org.uk/advice/esuom50/chapter/Key-points-from-the-evidence (accessed 17 July 2017).

- Vale C, Burdett S, Rydzewska L, *et al.* Addition of docetaxel or bisphosphonates to standard of care in men with localized or metastatic, hormone-sensitive prostate cancer: a systematic review and meta-analyses of aggregate data. *Lancet Oncol* 2016; 17: 243–56.

16 Integrated Care When Cancer Is Diagnosed in Pregnancy

Richard Simcock, Pete Wallroth

Case history

A 40-year-old woman in her second pregnancy was diagnosed at 24 weeks' gestation with a clinically node-positive grade 3 invasive ductal breast cancer measuring 6.5 cm in diameter. It had initially been thought to be a blocked milk duct. The tumour was oestrogen receptor (ER)-, progesterone receptor (PR)- and human epidermal growth factor receptor 2 (HER2)-negative. On the basis of size, neoadjuvant chemotherapy was recommended. Staging was performed with a liver ultrasound and a chest radiograph. Chemotherapy with fluorouracil, epirubicin and cyclophosphamide was commenced. There was close liaison with obstetric services.

The chemotherapy was well tolerated and there was clinical evidence of response with tumour shrinkage. A planned induction of labour took place at 37 weeks' gestation, 3 weeks after completion of four cycles of chemotherapy. Labour was induced with a prostaglandin vaginal tablet. The delivery was uncomplicated. The patient gave birth to a healthy baby son weighing 3.7 kg. The baby was fed with donor breast milk.

Shortly after the birth the patient restarted chemotherapy with planned docetaxel treatment. The breast tumour was barely palpable at this point. The chemotherapy was associated with significant fatigue and nausea and she required prolonged bed rest. She began to suffer migraines for the first time.

Following her seventh chemotherapy session the patient became very unwell and was admitted to hospital with severe migraines, dehydration, sickness and blurred vision and a Glasgow Coma Score of 13. Contrast-enhanced MRI showed meningeal thickening consistent with leptomeningeal disease. The diagnosis was confirmed on subsequent lumbar puncture. There was some brief improvement with dexamethasone but then further and rapid deterioration. After a 12 day admission she was transferred to her local hospice. She died there peacefully 3 days later surrounded by her family. Her son was 2 months old and her daughter was 3 years old. The patient and her family were supported throughout the process by the charity Mummy's Star and a named midwife and breast care nurse.

How does the treatment of pregnancy-associated breast cancer differ from standard care?

How should obstetric/antenatal services and oncology services combine in these cases?

How can charities or third sector partners help in cases of pregnancy-associated cancer?

What opportunities are there to collect and share data on these relatively rare cases?

How does the treatment of pregnancy-associated breast cancer differ from standard care?

The incidence of pregnancy-associated breast cancer is rising due to the trend for later pregnancies and the increasing incidence of breast cancer with age (53% of all live births in England and Wales in 2015 were to mothers aged 30 and over).[1] There is European consensus guidance for the treatment of pregnancy-associated breast cancer:[2] as no randomized data were available, evidence was taken from retrospective datasets, which appear to demonstrate that pregnancy does not worsen cancer prognosis.[3]

It has been suggested that the hormonal changes of pregnancy and the lactational breast changes may be important drivers of the disease.[4] The diagnosis of breast cancer may be delayed because the changes caused by the cancer are mistaken for normal lactational changes in the breast or (as in this case) a blocked duct. Non-ionizing imaging (MRI, ultrasound) or reduced dose (chest radiograph) should be used if deemed necessary. Gadolinium should not be used during MRI. Surgery appears safe, but blue dye should not be used at sentinel node biopsy. Reconstruction should be delayed due to lactational asymmetry. Subsequent treatment is determined by the trimester of the pregnancy. In the first trimester, chemotherapy should be avoided. In the second and third trimesters, chemotherapy may be delivered at standard doses. Standard antiemetics including steroids and 5-HT$_3$ antagonists may be used. Trastuzumab should be avoided due to an association with oligohydramnios. Tamoxifen should be avoided in pregnancy. It would be rare to offer radiotherapy during pregnancy due to concerns around fetal dose. It may be possible (due to inverse-square law) to deliver treatment in the first trimester when the fetus is small and distant from the breast.[5]

How should obstetric/antenatal services and oncology services combine in these cases?

Early collaboration and communication between obstetric, oncology and primary care teams are an essential component of care.[6] Midwives and breast care nurses should collaborate to act as key workers for the patient. Early discussion should include reassurance to the patient and her family that the pregnancy can usually progress safely to term.

Some patients may wish to consider termination of pregnancy in the context of their cancer diagnosis. These patients should be counselled carefully by both oncology and obstetric teams that with good coordination both cancer and antenatal care can be delivered appropriately. Patients should be reassured that cohort studies have shown no adverse impact on longer term child health after exposure to chemotherapy *in utero*.[7]

Timing of delivery is an important point of discussion for the patient and the team. Fetal health improves with every week of gestation, and delivery should occur as close to term as possible. If full gestation dates fall during the chemotherapy schedule then a planned induction past the chemotherapy nadir is sensible. In the rare cases in which an elective caesarean section is felt to be necessary earlier in the pregnancy then steroids may be used to accelerate fetal lung development.[8]

How can charities or third sector partners help in cases of pregnancy-associated cancer?

This was a very isolating time for the patient and her family not only because of her age but because of the timing in the pregnancy. The family had never heard of cases of cancer being diagnosed let alone treated in pregnancy before and they feared for the survival of their baby.

On diagnosis the patient was signposted by her breast care nurse to the charity Mummy's Star, among others. Mummy's Star (www.mummysstar.org) is a specialist charity established to support women diagnosed with cancer in or around a pregnancy. By connecting with the charity and therefore being in contact with other mothers in the UK and Ireland, the patient did not feel alone and was able to share her thoughts and fears with others who had been in a similar situation and learn of their experience during pregnancy. Service users of Mummy's Star cite the peer support as an invaluable service, as the cancer otherwise deprives them of the normal, happy experience of an evolving pregnancy. Similar organizations exist overseas, such as Hope for Two (www.hopefortwo.org) in the USA.

The patient was unable to breastfeed her son, as she had with her first child, because of chemotherapy. Mummy's Star were able to intervene and advocate on her behalf and support her midwifery team in securing donor breast milk from a regional milk bank. Milk was couriered to the house each week by a local blood courier service. This handed a significant amount of control back to the mother.

The patient's husband had needed to take much more than his allowed paternity leave from work and the couple were beginning to struggle financially. Through the grant support programme at Mummy's Star they were able to reclaim some of the lost expenditure, which eased pressures. Mummy's Star also referred the family to the home support charity Home-Start (www.home-start.org.uk), which following a home visit matched a volunteer who offered weekly visits for a few hours' assistance with domestic chores. This eased the pressure on the family.

Mummy's Star was founded after the death of its CEO's wife from pregnancy-associated breast cancer. The CEO was therefore able to further support the patient's husband in bereavement by connecting him with other widowers of a similar age. This peer support proved invaluable to helping him and his children come to terms with their loss, culminating in a residential weekend where they were able to have a holiday break with others who had had a similar experience, thus reducing a significant amount of isolation. In addition, Mummy's Star was able to support the family with advice on entitlements such as Widowed Parent's Allowance and further financial support.

In the palliative care setting midwives maintained contact with the family to help the patient build bonds with her baby and to ensure good feeding. This continuity was valuable at a time of significant and rapid change.

What opportunities are there to collect and share data on these relatively rare cases?

It is important to collect data on outcomes of pregnancy-associated breast cancer for both mother and child in the absence of randomized data. Long-term childhood outcome data are particularly sparse. Cancer centres or obstetric units may voluntarily register with the International Network on Cancer, Infertility and Pregnancy (www.cancerinpregnancy.org). This register collects data from across Europe. Centres contributing data to the registry are considered research partners for the use of the data.

Conclusion and learning points

- Pregnancy-associated breast cancer may be treated with minor modifications to standard protocols and has outcomes consistent with breast cancer of similar stage in non-pregnant patients.

- Close liaison with obstetric services and midwives should permit delivery as close to pregnancy full term as possible to ensure optimum fetal health.

- Mummy's Star is a charity which can help families coping with pregnancy-associated breast cancer by providing peer support, financial aid and specialist knowledge.

- Patients should be reassured that there is no evidence of developmental abnormalities in children exposed to chemotherapy *in utero*.

References

1 Office for National Statistics (2016). *Births by parents' characteristics in England and Wales: 2015.* Available from:
www.ons.gov.uk/peoplepopulationandcommunity/birthsdeathsandmarriages/
livebirths/bulletins/birthsbyparentscharacteristicsinenglandandwales/2015 (accessed February 2017).

2 Amant F, Deckers S, Van Calsteren K, *et al.* Breast cancer in pregnancy: recommendations of an international consensus meeting. *Eur J Cancer* 2010; 46: 3158–68.

3 Amant F, Von Minckwitz G, Han SN, *et al.* Prognosis of women with primary breast cancer diagnosed during pregnancy: results from an international collaborative study. *J Clin Oncol* 2013; 31: 2532–9.

4 McCready J, Arendt LM, Glover E, *et al.* Pregnancy-associated breast cancers are driven by differences in adipose stromal cells present during lactation. *Breast Cancer Res* 2014; 16: R2.

5 Kal HB, Struikmans H. Radiotherapy during pregnancy: fact and fiction. *Lancet Oncol* 2005; 6: 328–33.

6 Royal College of Obstetricians and Gynaecologists (2011). *Pregnancy and breast cancer. Green-top guideline no. 12.* Available from: www.rcog.org.uk/en/guidelines-research-services/guidelines/gtg12 (accessed February 2017).

7 Murthy RK, Theriault RL, Barnett CM. Outcomes of children exposed *in utero* to chemotherapy for breast cancer. *Breast Cancer Res* 2014; 16: 500.

8 Cordeiro CN, Gemignani MD. Breast cancer in pregnancy: avoiding fetal harm when maternal treatment is necessary. *Breast J* 2017; 23: 200–5.

17 Integrated Care in the Treatment of Head and Neck Malignancy

Siobhan Morrison, Andrew Fishburn, Anne Carter, Rachel Hewitson, Katy Everson, Muthiah Sivaramalingam

Case history

A 62-year-old woman presented with an 8 week history of worsening sore throat. She had a medical history of migraine and primary sclerosing cholangitis. She was a non-smoker, drank alcohol occasionally and had a performance status of zero.

She was diagnosed with moderately differentiated squamous cell carcinoma of the hypopharynx, T2N0M0. To attempt organ preservation, the proposed management plan was radical chemoradiotherapy (65 Gy in 30 fractions and weekly cisplatin). The multidisciplinary team did not consider localized resection an appropriate option. Before starting treatment the patient underwent dental, nutritional, and speech and language assessments; a gastrostomy tube was also inserted.

During treatment she developed typical side effects of oral mucositis, odynophagia and subsequent dysphagia. Her weight decreased and she became dependent on the gastrostomy tube for all her nutritional and fluid requirements.

Two weeks after completion of treatment she was reviewed by a clinical nurse specialist, dietitian, and speech and language therapist. They advised introducing liquids orally and progressing to a soft diet as soon as possible. The patient struggled with this due to ongoing mucositis and pain. At 6 weeks her symptoms were improving but she still could not swallow. Flexible nasendoscopy showed minimal oedema, but videofluoroscopy demonstrated a stricture and aspiration. An MRI scan 12 weeks after treatment showed a good response and no visible residual tumour.

Improvement over subsequent months was slow, however, and the patient remained completely dysphagic. Several failed attempts were made by ENT and interventional radiology to dilate the cricopharyngeal stricture. An MRI scan 12 months after treatment showed ongoing, significant oedema, and the patient was referred for a second opinion regarding stricture dilation. With successful serial balloon dilations over several months, slow improvements in her swallow were observed. Videofluoroscopy performed by the speech and language therapist 18 months after treatment showed the patient was no longer aspirating and could safely swallow all consistencies. After a further 6 months of intensive support from the dietitian, speech and language therapist, clinical nurse specialist, oncologist and ENT surgeon she was able to have her gastrostomy tube removed, 2 years after completion of treatment. She remained free of disease recurrence and was able to maintain her weight with oral nutrition and continue on routine follow-up.

What was the goal of cancer treatment for this patient?

What is the evidence base for her treatment options?

What interventions help maintain nutritional intake during chemoradiotherapy for head and neck cancer patients?

What head and neck radiotherapy complications can occur and how are they managed?

How did an integrated care team benefit her during and after treatment?

What was the goal of cancer treatment for this patient?

The goals of treatment for a T2N0M0 squamous cell carcinoma of the hypopharynx are cure and organ function preservation, providing the patient is fit enough to undergo concurrent chemoradiotherapy. The side effects expected with radical treatment are substantial and often lead to deterioration or complete loss of swallow function. Steps must be taken to maintain nutritional support during treatment. The aim is then for the patient to return to normal swallow function as soon as possible after treatment. If return of function is slow, as in this case, investigations are needed to identify a treatable problem such as a stricture.

What is the evidence base for her treatment options?

Concurrent chemoradiotherapy for the treatment of unresectable head and neck squamous cell cancers is well established. The concurrent use of single-agent cisplatin with radiotherapy has been shown to be superior to radiotherapy alone, and the additional toxicities are manageable.[1-3] Combination chemotherapy regimens have been investigated and show superior response rates but no improvement in survival.[4] Weekly cisplatin is preferred, as it has been shown to be as effective as 3 weekly regimens but with less toxicity.[5]

The French Meta-Analysis of Chemotherapy in Head and Neck Cancer (MACH-NC) Collaborative Group carried out a meta-analysis of the impact on survival when chemotherapy was added to locoregional treatment.[1,2] Sixty-three trials between 1965 and 1993 were analysed and showed an absolute survival benefit of around 4% (36% from 32%) at 5 years in favour of chemotherapy. The heterogeneity of the trials meant these results were interpreted with caution. The MACH-NC update in 2000 included the additional randomized trials between 1994 and 2000 and confirmed the benefit of chemotherapy: 4.5% absolute survival benefit at 5 years. In particular, the benefit of concomitant chemotherapy over induction chemotherapy was seen, with a hazard ratio of 0.81 and an absolute survival benefit of 6.5% at 5 years.

The Head and Neck Intergroup trial was an American multi-institutional phase III randomized trial comprising 295 patients enrolled between 1992 and 1999.[3] Unresectable head and neck squamous cell cancer patients were randomly assigned to receive radiotherapy alone (control arm A), radiotherapy with concurrent cisplatin on days 1, 22 and 43 (arm B), or a split radiotherapy course and three cycles of concurrent infusional fluorouracil and cisplatin (arm C). Median follow-up was 41 months and the 3 year projected overall survival was 23% for arm A compared with 37% for arm B ($p=0.014$) and 27% for arm C (p-value not significant). Grades 3–5 toxicity in arm A was 51% compared with 89% in arm B ($p<0.001$) and 77% in arm C ($p<0.001$). The increase in toxicities with concurrent chemotherapy was not surprising, but the hospitals participating in the study reported they were very manageable.

What interventions help maintain nutritional intake during chemoradiotherapy for head and neck cancer patients?

Patients undergoing chemoradiotherapy for head and neck cancer experience significant side effects that affect nutritional intake, including mucositis and dysphagia,[6] loss of taste/taste changes, thick oropharyngeal secretions and xerostomia. Early nutritional intervention is key in maintaining nutritional intake during treatment. At our centre all patients have a nutritional assessment in the pretreatment clinic undertaken by a specialist dietitian. Intervention aims to improve, maintain or reduce decline in nutritional status of patients who have malnutrition or who may be at risk of malnutrition. Patients such as this woman undergoing chemoradiotherapy at the Royal Preston Hospital have the choice of prophylactic gastrostomy or rescue nasogastric tube. The benefits and risks of the two options are explored prior to treatment and the patient then makes a decision about which strategy to follow.

Nutritional surveillance is essential for patients undergoing treatment,[7] and they receive weekly monitoring of weight and nutritional intake by a specialist dietitian during the course of chemoradiotherapy. Appropriate advice is given on how to meet the deficit of nutritional intake when the treatment side effects commence and progress; emphasis is placed on maintaining oral intake for as long as possible with the aim of retaining swallow function and reducing post-treatment dependence on a feeding tube.[8] Appropriate supplementation with food fortification, sip feeds, bolus feeds and pump feeding are employed to meet nutritional requirements when required.

What head and neck radiotherapy complications can occur and how are they managed?

Acute radiotherapy side effects tend to develop after about 2 weeks of treatment. Tiredness is a generic side effect with all radiotherapy and other toxicities are then localized to the treated area. Externally, the skin within the radiotherapy field can become red, itchy and painful. The skin can break down and often needs barrier creams and dressings. Radiation skin reaction can last for up to 4 weeks after treatment. Patients are advised to cover up in the sun, not use perfumed soaps or creams, wear loose-fitting clothes and not to shave.

Internally, the mouth and throat can become very sore with the development of mucositis. Various mouth washes and analgesia, often morphine-based, are used and any infections are promptly treated. Owing to the pain, patients struggle to swallow, not only nutrition and fluids but also their own saliva. Secretions can build up and be quite distressing. Gastrostomy tubes, placed prior to treatment, are used when a patient is not meeting nutritional requirements or cannot swallow medications. If a tube is not pre-emptively placed, nasogastric feeding may be required to support the patient through the treatment.

Radiotherapy can affect the salivary glands, leading to a dry mouth, causing further difficulties with eating and talking. Patients are advised to sip water frequently; the effects can take months to improve. Long-term saliva production often never returns to normal.

The development of post-radiotherapy strictures is a late effect that can require recurrent dilations, as in this case. Other late effects include development of a stiff and sore neck due to muscle damage, neurological arm symptoms due to brachial plexus damage, and increased risk of stroke due to vessel damage in the irradiated field. Tooth decay is a late effect and patients are advised about maintaining good dental hygiene during and after treatment; they also undergo a dental assessment prior to treatment so that any necessary work can be carried out.

How did an integrated care team benefit her during and after treatment?

Integrated care before, during and after treatment enables combined appointment times and seamless working. There is much interlinking of roles in managing the side effects of treatment: by working together the oncologist, dietitian, speech and language therapist and clinical nurse specialist provide a holistic service. After meeting her oncologist and consenting to treatment, the patient attended a standard pretreatment multidisciplinary clinic (comprising a dietitian, a speech and language therapist and a clinical nurse specialist) and was counselled on the treatment logistics and side effects so she knew what to expect; she received a holistic needs assessment, as well as swallowing and nutritional assessments. Weekly treatment reviews were carried out by the oncologist alongside the dietitian and speech and language therapist. The same dietitian, speech and language therapist and clinical nurse specialist team reviewed the patient within 2 weeks of completing treatment. They offered symptom management, swallowing strategies and a nutritional plan to support progress towards removal of the gastrostomy tube. The benefits of multidisciplinary post-treatment support clinics providing psychological support and nutritional or functional (swallowing) support are described in the literature.[9-11] As the patient's side effects were slow to improve, she continued to be followed up at frequent intervals by the integrated care team. When they were not able to progress her from being dependent on the gastrostomy tube, the ENT and interventional radiology teams were called upon to diagnose and manage her stricture.

Conclusion and learning points

- Chemoradiotherapy is the radical treatment of choice for organ preservation in inoperable early-stage head and neck squamous cell carcinoma.

- Concurrent weekly cisplatin confers improved overall survival compared with radiotherapy alone and is less toxic than 3 weekly or combined chemotherapy regimens.

- Head and neck chemoradiotherapy side effects have a significant impact on quality of life and require medical intervention and psychological support to ensure patients complete their treatment.

- Swallow function and nutritional intake require careful monitoring and support, before, during and after treatment, by multidisciplinary specialists.

- Post-radiotherapy strictures can be difficult to manage, but improvements in swallow function with recurrent dilation can lead to reinstatement of oral intake and removal of a feeding tube even up to 2 years after treatment.

References

1 Pignon JP, Bourhis J, Domenge C, Designe L. Chemotherapy added to locoregional treatment for head and neck squamous-cell carcinoma: three meta-analyses of updated individual data. *Lancet* 2000; 355: 949–55.

2 Pignon JP, le Maître A, Maillard E, *et al*. Meta-analysis of chemotherapy in head and neck cancer (MACH-NC): an update on 93 randomised trials and 17,346 patients. *Radiother Oncol* 2009; 92: 4–14.

3 Adelstein DJ, Li Y, Adams GL, *et al*. An intergroup phase III comparison of standard radiation therapy and two schedules of concurrent chemoradiotherapy in patients with unresectable squamous cell head and neck cancer. *J Clin Oncol* 2003; 21: 92–8.

4 Jacobs C, Lyman G, Velez-García E, *et al*. A phase III randomized study comparing cisplatin and fluorouracil as single agents and in combination for advanced squamous cell carcinoma of the head and neck. *J Clin Oncol* 1992; 10: 257–63.

5   Melotek JM, Cooper BT, Koshy M, *et al.* Weekly versus every-three-weeks platinum-based chemoradiation regimens for head and neck cancer. *J Otolaryngol Head Neck Surg* 2016; 45: 62.

6   Franzcr JC, Poon W, McPhee N, *et al.* Prospective study of percutaneous endoscopic gastrostomy tubes versus nasogastric tubes for enteral feeding in patients with head and neck cancer undergoing (chemo)radiation. *Head Neck* 2009; 31: 867–76.

7   Ehrsson YT, Langius-Eklöf A, Laurell G. Nutritional surveillance and weight loss in head and neck cancer patients. *Support Care Cancer* 2012; 20: 757–65.

8   Bhayani MK, Hutcheson KA, Barringer DA, *et al.* Gastrostomy tube placement in patients with oropharyngeal carcinoma treated with radiotherapy or chemoradiotherapy: factors affecting placement and dependence. *Head Neck* 2013; 35: 1634–40.

9   Gould L, Lewis S. Care of head and neck cancer patients with swallowing difficulties. *Br J Nurs* 2006; 15: 1091–6.

10 Hewett J, Howland D. The benefits of a nurse and dietician-led follow-up clinic in head and neck cancer. *Cancer Nurs Pract* 2009; 8: 23–7.

11 van der Meulen IC, May AM, Ros WJ, *et al.* One-year effect of a nurse-led psychosocial intervention on depressive symptoms in patients with head and neck cancer: a randomized controlled trial. *Oncologist* 2013; 18: 336–44.

Further reading

• Chen AM, Li BQ, Lau DH, *et al.* Evaluating the role of prophylactic gastrostomy tube placement prior to definitive chemoradiotherapy for head and neck cancer. *Int J Radiat Oncol Biol Phys* 2010; 78: 1026–32.

• Harrison LB, Sessions RB, Kies MS, eds. *Head and neck cancer: a multidisciplinary approach.* 4th rev. ed. Philadelphia, PA: Lippincott Williams & Wilkins, Wolters Kluwer, 2014.

• Wall LR, Ward EC, Cartmill B, *et al.* Physiological changes to the swallowing mechanism following (chemo)radiotherapy for head and neck cancer: a systematic review. *Dysphagia* 2013; 28: 481–93.

18 Vulvovaginal Pain after Breast Cancer Treatment

Josie Butcher

Case history

A 41-year-old woman presented 36 months after a diagnosis of grade 3 invasive ductal carcinoma: oestrogen receptor (ER)-positive, progesterone receptor (PR)-positive, human epidermal growth factor receptor 2 (HER2)-negative, lymph node-positive. Initial surgery was a lumpectomy, followed by mastectomy, chemotherapy and radiotherapy. She had been considering breast reconstruction and had been taking tamoxifen for 2 years with the expectation that it would be needed for a further 8 years.

She had returned to work but reduced her hours to half time so that she could spend more time with her young children. She is married and describes herself as being in a loving, caring relationship with good emotional support throughout her illness.

Over the previous 6 months she had mentioned to a number of health professionals that she had little interest in engaging in 'intimate relations' with her husband. Discussions with her team focused on diet, exercise and developing a good sleep pattern, and she felt they had looked at body image with her as part of her work-up for breast reconstruction. She is supremely grateful for the quality of life (QOL), and possibly the length of life, she is now able to have. She did not understand why she found it difficult to engage intimately with her husband: she did not seem to want sex, nor became aroused, and did not know why she found penetration so painful. She worried about the lack of what was previously a good sexual life and felt that eventually her husband would find a new partner. She was getting increasingly anxious but felt she could not ask more from a team who had given so much and who she perceived would find this problem frivolous.

When the oncology registrar elicited her concerns and took a full sexual history, the patient described two problems: lack of interest and vaginal pain likened to having 'razor blades' in her vagina. Initial interest in resuming sexual activity stopped when penetration pain was severe, leading to withdrawal from sexual contact, then withdrawal from affectionate contact because of anxiety that any contact might lead to sex. She recognized her avoidance and lack of communication with her husband, reporting that they now go to bed at different times to avoid contact.

Her difficulties also affected other areas of her life. Along with fatigue, the increasing vulvovaginal pain had stopped her from dancing, which led to withdrawal from her friendship group; she had become socially isolated, which affected her self-confidence. She reported discomfort when simply sitting at her computer; she had sought, and tried, online advice. She remained active as a school mum and felt it critically important to spend as much time as she could with her children.

She clearly described a good sexual history prior to diagnosis and even through the initial process of treatments, reporting no previous problems with desire and interest, arousal and orgasm. Examination revealed atrophic vaginitis.

Do sexual problems affect many cancer patients, and why are they such a big problem?

Why do cancer patients find it difficult to talk about sexual problems?

How should you proceed with this patient?

What examinations and/or investigations are appropriate?

What treatment options are available?

Do sexual problems affect many cancer patients, and why are they such a big problem?

The aim of this case study is to offer a framework for all healthcare professionals to assist them to open conversations about sexual problems and offer help. The discussions suggested apply to all patients whatever their sex, sexual orientation or sexual problems.

Sexual difficulties following cancer are well recognized. Two pivotal Macmillan Cancer Support surveys give a good insight into patient need: 43% of patients reported that their sexual life had suffered and 26% had worries about their relationship.[1,2] Patients cited the change of role of partner into carer, body image issues and mental health concerns. Prostate Cancer UK and others have made similar findings (personal communication, 2010). Patients have reported that they would like health professionals to ask about their sexual life, but many health professionals say they find such conversations difficult, and feel embarrassed and out of control.[3,4] Health professionals identified that for control they needed to know: whether to ask, when to ask, how to ask, what to ask, and what to do with the answers.[4] NICE guidelines along with a number of Department of Health collaborative documents recognize the importance of being able to discuss sexual issues.[5] Glantz et al.[6] found that divorce following cancer was more likely to occur after a brain tumour, but in all cancers it was far more likely if the patient was female.

Part of the concerns we have as health professionals in opening conversations is that for all of us this is a private area of our life and hence not an area we usually discuss with others. It is as difficult for the health professional to start the conversation as it is for the patient to respond.

Why do cancer patients find it difficult to talk about sexual problems?

Bancroft's research into sexual behaviour confirms that sex is seen as a very private part of life that is vulnerable to societal and media attitudes.[7] Bancroft studied the concept of socially desirable answering by patients and, hence, patient disempowerment.[8] How can patients ask for what is seen as a lifestyle option by many, when they should just be satisfied that they have been given back their life? Current evidence on metastatic breast cancer patients from McClelland suggests the importance of QOL.[9] Although hers was a small qualitative study, the findings suggest that breast cancer treatment should include discussion about future sexual life. Similar studies are being conducted in other cancers.[4,10] Both patients and health professionals regard the barriers to discussion to be embarrassment, anxiety and loss of control.

How should you proceed with this patient?

Do not assume or rely on the assessments of other colleagues, but make your own assessment, taking a history of the presenting complaint and a sexual history. The linear model of sexual function shows the sequence of separate physiological events that illustrate good sexual function.[11] Each element – desire, arousal, orgasm and resolution – can be affected by the disease process and/or the anatomical and physiological damage caused by surgical intervention or treatment. Each physiological event works independently of the others and demands an intact anatomy and neurological, vascular and hormonal systems. Remember to look beyond patients whose surgery and treatments affect the genital systems directly, as all patients can have sexual consequences of their disease and treatments.

Once a thorough history has been taken, other areas should be considered for investigation. Weeks and Gambescia[12] used an integrated biopsychosocial model of assessment and care (Figure 18.1),[4] which is essential if we are to consider the full impact of sexual difficulties. Considerations include medical history and treatments; the partner's needs; the sense of sexual self, which offers information on the patient's vulnerabilities as well as on the religious and cultural needs;[11] relationship(s) and current difficulties; and the patient's social constructs. The latter includes the workplace, social life, hobbies, family life in general and how the problems impact all areas of life, as in the present case. The internationally recognized *Diagnostic and statistical manual of mental disorders (DSM-5)*[13] is preferred for its specificity with regard to the physiology of the sexual response.

What examinations and/or investigations are appropriate?

It is important that the oncology team examine the area of concern irrespective of the primary diagnosis. In our patient's case, the breast area had frequently been examined, but very little attention had been paid to her vaginal pain, leading to anxiety that the cancer had spread. Examination and investigation should be offered in the same way that vaginal bleeding is investigated in postmenopausal women or in women taking tamoxifen. If examination reveals atrophic vaginitis then reassurance can be offered. Owing to the severity of her pain, the patient

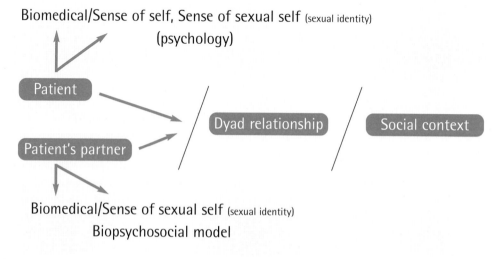

Figure 18.1 Assessment using integrated therapy (adapted from Weeks and Gambescia[12]).

did not feel reassured that it was just a side effect of the tamoxifen. Her lack of self-confidence and social withdrawal suggested the need for a mental health assessment.

What treatment options are available?

The patient agreed to focus on realistic goals that included psychoeducation and reduction of vaginal pain, working towards reintroducing intimacy, including exploring vaginal penetration.

The PLISSIT model describes levels of therapeutic intervention (Figure 18.2).[14] Permission for both the patient and health professional to open the conversation to address sexual difficulties is crucial.[4,6,15] Once limited information has been elicited, psychoeducation explores the impact of the problem on the patient's biopsychosocial life (Figure 18.1). Understanding the physiological change using simple schematic diagrams of the vulvovaginal area and vaginal wall helped the patient understand, or 'normalize', her difficulty, which increased her confidence. Exploring the impact of sexual problems on her relationship and recognizing the loss incurred by this, for herself as well as the perceived loss for her partner, led to cognitive reframing of her thoughts. Exploring her sense of sexual self,[11] motherhood, her work role and friendships enabled marked changes in her understanding and a reduction in her anxiety. For some patients this is enough; however, it is important in a partnership to attempt couple discussions and mutual understanding.

Specific suggestions for all oncology patients include: psychoeducation, relaxation programmes, mindfulness, body ownership and body awareness (mind and body working together), as well as help relating to specific sexual difficulties. For men, solution-focused products for erectile dysfunction are helpful (see Chapter 14, Table 14.2). Positive steps for female patients are exploration of body ownership, body image and reasons for avoidance of intimacy, as well as treatment options for painful areas. If the woman avoids touching the perineum, use of aqueous cream as a soap substitute (requires rinsing off to prevent skin thinning) or Dermal products, applied by hand, with showers preferable to bathing, retains moisture in the skin. A simple moisturizer as well as a daily lubricant to the introitus maintains 'vulval care'. Good lubricants, both aqueous and oil-based, are available; however, oil-based lubricants degrade most condoms and need to be avoided if condom use is essential. Within a month of this simple vulval care programme, patients feel more comfortable sitting, walking, exercising and wearing trousers, thus taking back ownership of the area of pain. Viewing the perineum in a mirror and charting areas of discomfort using a cotton bud furthers ownership. Teaching pelvic floor relaxation enables the patient to learn to control vaginal muscle spasms, an automatic response to any vaginal pain condition; control is needed before desensitization techniques using graded dilators can be

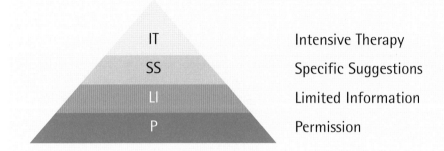

Figure 18.2 The PLISSIT model: what to do with the answers and when.[14]

introduced. A good lubricant to reduce friction gives the patient the confidence and ability to control vaginal pain. The patient then learns what is possible in terms of penetration.

Successful reintroduction of intimacy needs the consent and understanding of both partners. Using body awareness, focusing on body sensations, allows the mind and body to work together, staying in the moment and learning to shut out performance anxiety: in this case, 'nothing's going to happen; it's going to hurt'. A typical sensate focus programme with the giving and receiving of touch, initially non-sexual, moving to exploratory touch and then to genital stimulation, can be successful. A ban on penetration and understanding the necessity of this are crucial to creating an atmosphere of trust. Couples gain improved communication, and often find themselves progressing to sexual stimulation without penetration. Improved communication leads to the development of foreplay, which may include the introduction of vibration if needed. Development of frictionless penetration following the desensitization programme offers recognition that sometimes it is easily possible but at other times it is very difficult. If sexual frequency is high the vagina may at times need to be 'rested'.

All the above treatments can be carried out by health professionals in the hospital and dealt with through training, supervision support and networking. Patients who require more help can be identified for appropriate referral.

References

1 Macmillan Cancer Support (2006). *Worried sick: the emotional impact of cancer.* Available from:
www.macmillan.org.uk/documents/getinvolved/campaigns/campaigns/impact_of_cancer_english.pdf (accessed 3 July 2017).

2 Macmillan Cancer Support. *It's no life: living with long term effects of cancer.* London: Macmillan Cancer Support, 2009.

3 Hopwood P, Swindle R, Cawthorn A, Richardson L. Audit results: nurse–patient communication about sexual concerns. Poster presented at: Cancer and Sexuality Interest Group, Christie Hospital NHS Foundation Trust, 2006.

4 Butcher J, Dobson C, Atkinson A, *et al.* Sex and cancer: opening difficult therapeutic conversations and challenging assumptions using design activism-language outside the comfort zone. *Sex Relat Ther* 2016; 31: 493–509.

5 National Institute for Health and Care Excellence (2012). *Patient experience in adult NHS services: improving the experience of care for people using adult NHS services.* Available from: http://guidance.nice.org.uk/cg138 (accessed 3 July 2017).

6 Glantz MJ, Chamberlain MC, Liu Q, *et al.* Gender disparity in the rate of partner abandonment in patients with serious medical illness. *Cancer* 2009; 115: 5237–42.

7 Bancroft J, ed. *Researching sexual behavior.* Indianapolis, IN: Kinsey Institute for Research in Sex, Gender, and Reproduction; Indiana University Press, 1997.

8 Crowne DP, Marlowe D. A new scale of social desirability independent of psychopathology. *J Consult Psychol* 1960; 24: 349–54.

9 McClelland SI. 'I wish I'd known': patients' suggestions for supporting sexual quality of life after diagnosis with metastatic breast cancer. *Sex Relat Ther* 2016; 31: 414–31.

10 O'Brien R, Rose P, Campbell C, *et al.* I wish I'd told them: a qualitative study examining the unmet psychosexual needs of prostate cancer patients during follow-up after treatment. *Patient Educ Couns* 2011; 84: 200–7.

11 Butcher J. Female sexual problems 1: loss of desire – what about the fun? In: Tomlinson JM,
ed. *ABC of sexual health.* 2nd ed. Oxford: Blackwell, 2005; 21–4.

12 Weeks GR, Gambescia N. *Hypoactive sexual desire: integrating sex and couple therapy.* New
York, NY: Norton, 2002.

13 American Psychiatric Association. *Diagnostic and statistical manual of mental disorders (DSM-
5).* 5th ed. Arlington, VA: American Psychiatric Publishing, 2013.

14 Annon JS. The PLISSIT model: a proposed conceptual scheme for the behavioral treatment of
sexual problems. *J Sex Educ Ther* 1976; 2.

15 Gordon P. The contribution of sexology to contemporary sexuality education. *Sex Marital
Ther* 1994; 9: 171–80.

Further reading

* Department of Health (2010). *Equity and excellence: liberating the NHS.* Available from:
  www.gov.uk/government/uploads/system/uploads/attachment_data/file/213823/dh_117794.
  pdf (accessed 3 July 2017).

* Department of Health (2013). *Updated NHS constitution published.* Available from:
  www.england.nhs.uk/2013/03/26/nhs-constitution (accessed 3 July 2017).

* Department of Health, Macmillan Cancer Support, NHS Improvement. *Living with and
  beyond cancer: taking action to improve outcomes.* London: Department of Health, 2013.

* Jun EY, Kim S, Chang SB, *et al.* The effect of a sexual life reframing program on marital
  intimacy, body image, and sexual function among breast cancer survivors. *Cancer Nurs* 2011;
  34: 142–9.

* Panjary M, Bell RJ, Davies SR. Sexual function after breast cancer. *J Sex Med* 2011; 8: 294–
  302.

* Papadopoulos L (2010). *Sexualisation of young people. Review.* Available from:
  http://dera.ioe.ac.uk/10738/1/sexualisation-young-people.pdf (accessed 3 July 2017).

* Tathanhlong L, McGuffin M, Bristow B. Exploring healthcare professional's comfort level and
  self-assessed competency on providing care to young breast cancer patients. *J Med Imaging
  Radiat Sci* 2014; 45: 171.

19 Use of Patient-Reported Outcome Measures to Enhance Follow-Up after Germ Cell Tumour Treatment

Oana C. Lindner, Dulani Ranatunge, Dan Stark

Case history

A 44-year-old man presented to primary care with left scrotal ache and a left testicular lump on self-examination. Approximately 1 month later he underwent inguinal orchidectomy. Histological examination revealed a stage I mixed germ cell tumour, pT1 (embryonal carcinoma with 10% seminoma), with negative margins. Tumour markers before surgery were alpha-fetoprotein (AFP) 3 μg/l (<7 μg/l), human chorionic gonadotrophin (hCG) <5 IU/l (<5 IU/l), lactate dehydrogenase (LDH) 8.2 μkat/l (<7.18 μkat/l). He had little relevant medical history.

After surgery his LDH level decreased to 6.26 μkat/l; histology results and radiological staging suggested that his treatment options included adjuvant chemotherapy (reducing the risk of recurrence to 4–5% but increasing the risk of early and late adverse effects) or surveillance (with an associated risk of relapse between 15% and 50%). Both result in identical long-term overall survival.

After multidisciplinary team (MDT) discussion and considering the balance of risks, the patient chose surveillance. He preferred to avoid chemotherapy unless absolutely necessary and wished to return to a normal day-to-day life as soon as possible. He understood he may have to return to chemotherapy later if relapse occurred and that it might be a longer course, especially if relapse was not detected promptly. Surveillance commenced later that month.

Appointments involved a blood investigation to monitor tumour markers, a chest X-ray or CT scan, and a short face-to-face appointment for clinical examination and discussion of results and of new or ongoing symptoms. The patient was in full-time employment, highly motivated and capable of managing his illness, but he needed to miss a day's work to attend appointments.

He was given an informed choice between standard follow-up and shared community follow-up, both described below. The patient chose community follow-up. He had a health promotion discussion, was provided with the log-in details for an online patient-reported outcome measures (PROMs) questionnaire (called QTool), and was given a bespoke follow-up schedule detailing the approximate dates of future assessments (Figure 19.1).

The patient has been in community follow-up for 20 months, reporting online his general health, back pain, testicular self-examination, and levels and causes of distress. His tumour markers and radiology indicated no activity from his cancer.

Enter month of completion of most recent treatment in blue box below, in the format
Jun-03

	Jul-15		
Patient name			
Date of birth			
Hospital number			
Interval of appointments (months)	Outpatient appointment date		Investigations required
1	Aug-15		AFP, hCG, LDH
2	Sep-15		AFP, hCG, LDH; CXR
3	Oct-15		AFP, hCG, LDH; CT scan
4	Nov-15		AFP, hCG, LDH; CXR
5	Dec-15		AFP, hCG, LDH
6	Jan-16		AFP, hCG, LDH; CXR
7	Feb-16		AFP, hCG, LDH
8	Mar-16		AFP, hCG, LDH; CXR
9	Apr-16		AFP, hCG, LDH
10	May-16		AFP, hCG, LDH; CXR
11	Jun-16		AFP, hCG, LDH
12	Jul-16		AFP, hCG, LDH; CT scan
14	Sep-16	Nurse-led	AFP, hCG, LDH
16	Nov-16	Nurse-led	AFP, hCG, LDH; CXR
18	Jan-17	Nurse-led	AFP, hCG, LDH
20	Mar-17	Nurse-led	AFP, hCG, LDH; CXR
22	May-17	Nurse-led	AFP, hCG, LDH
24	Jul-17	Nurse-led	AFP, hCG, LDH; CXR
27	Oct-17	Nurse-led	AFP, hCG, LDH
30	Jan-18	Nurse-led	AFP, hCG, LDH; CXR
33	Apr-18	Nurse-led	AFP, hCG, LDH
36	Jul-18	Nurse-led	AFP, hCG, LDH; CXR
42	Jan-19	Nurse-led	AFP, hCG, LDH; CXR
48	Jul-19	Nurse-led	AFP, hCG, LDH; CXR
54	Jan-20	Nurse-led	AFP, hCG, LDH
60	Jul-20	Nurse-led	AFP, hCG, LDH; CXR

Discharge at 5 years, or to long-term follow-up if aged up to 30th birthday at the point of
diagnosis (unless in a trial and protocol dictates otherwise)

Figure 19.1 Follow-up protocol for low-risk stage I non-seminomatous germ cell tumour (intense surveillance
programme). CXR, chest X-ray.

Eight QTool evaluations revealed no self-examination changes; however, they did reveal changes in other outcomes (Figure 19.2). Initially, QTool revealed poorer general health, mild back pain and increased emotional distress due to feelings of sadness, regret about the past, and inability to access spiritual support. Distress levels improved over 6 months; when elevated, discussion revealed that the main sources were surgical (discomfort in the inguinal scar/remaining testicle and back) and psychological (due to his present social context: fatigue, regret about the past, memory/concentration problems). Back pain reduced by the 5th month but increased in the 8th month. In parallel, the patient's general health decreased and distress levels increased (due to breathing difficulties and work issues). The patient was recalled to clinic and investigated but no relapse was found.

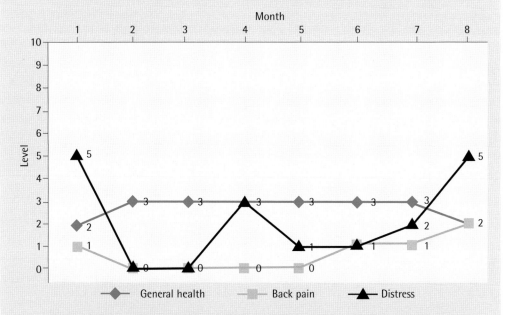

Figure 19.2 General health (0, very poor; 3, good), back pain (0, no back pain; 3, severe back pain) and distress (0, no distress; 10, very high level of distress). Note: higher scores on pain and distress indicate a poorer outcome, while higher scores on general health suggest a better outcome.

The patient is presently highly compliant and satisfied with community follow-up but is aware he can revert to standard follow-up at any time.

What is the evidence base for routine follow-up?

What key issues are addressed during follow-up, from a patient and a clinical perspective?

What are the benefits and challenges of standard follow-up?

What are the benefits and challenges of community follow-up?

How can online assessments of symptoms support community follow-up?

What are patients' opinions of online assessment?

What is the evidence base for routine follow-up?

Clinical monitoring and review are needed to identify cancer recurrence, to prevent or manage late effects and to provide reassurance.[1] Effective follow-up systems provide clinicians and patients with confidence during surveillance for resected stage I disease (despite the availability of a treatment to reduce that risk) and therefore minimize overtreatment and late effects. The risk of recurrence reduces over time, but relapse requires urgent intervention to maintain outcomes.[2] For instance, for stage I seminoma, after resection of the primary, management may include surveillance, chemotherapy or radiotherapy. Relapse rates vary from 8% to over 30% based on clinical risk groups and management,[3] but surgery alone has few late effects. If the management includes chemotherapy or radiotherapy, platinum-based treatments can result in ototoxicity, neuropathy and fertility issues, while bleomycin may lead to pulmonary toxicity. Psychological late effects management is required in the long term irrespective of clinical management;[4] hence, care after cancer needs to be holistic and pertain to relapse detection and wider patient needs.

Evidence-based follow-up is implemented for patients at St James's University Hospital, who are placed on one of 13 risk-stratified pathways (Figure 19.3) defined by disease stage and risk of relapse.[5,6] Each pathway defines the frequency and timing of investigations and outpatient appointments (Figure 19.4) for 3, 5 or 10 years after treatment. For our patient, the pathway involved frequent blood tests and clinical appointments ($n=26$), chest X-rays ($n=8$) and CT scans ($n=6$) over 5 years. In standard follow-up, all 26 appointments would have taken place in the specialist cancer centre, 15 miles from his home.

In community follow-up, patients are reminded by post (and/or email or text message) when an assessment is required and asked to arrange their blood test and chest X-ray within 7 days by any preferred competent NHS provider (i.e. GP practice, local district hospital, or, increasingly, at a supermarket). Within 14 days they should log on to QTool from any web-enabled device to complete a questionnaire on symptoms and distress that uses PROMs.

Clerical specialist MDT members retrieve investigation results for clinicians to review in their office. Even if there are no concerns about the tumour markers or radiology, no symptoms or concerns are reported online and there is no request from the patient for a face-to-face review, patients still meet their clinical team at St James's for a review of their CT scans at least once a year (for our patient, six times in 5 years). Patients can contact their clinical team directly via telephone or email about potential concerns between assessments.

What key issues are addressed during follow-up, from a patient and a clinical perspective?

The traditional clinical models for cancer follow-up focus on detection of recurrence (based on clinical examination and symptoms, tumour markers and radiological surveillance), and on monitoring acute and late adverse effects of treatment. The holistic approach to patient care during follow-up emphasizes the management of distress levels and the impact of cancer- and treatment-related late effects on the patient's life.[7,8] At present, assessing patient distress and emotional support usually falls to the clinical nurse specialist.

Patients value several aspects of follow-up: holistic assessments that take into account their wider needs, receiving timely results and reassurance after clinical investigations, being able to rely on specialist reviews of their physical status, and receiving specialist advice to manage late physical and psychological effects.[9,10]

What are the benefits and challenges of standard follow-up?

It has been shown that clinical examinations are not beneficial in detecting germ cell tumour

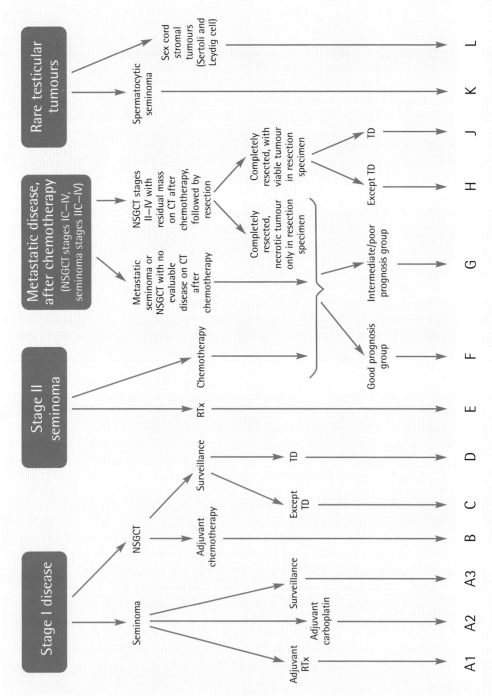

Figure 19.3 St James's University Hospital local germ cell tumour follow-up guidelines, showing 13 follow-up pathways (A1 to L) after treatment. NSGCT, non-seminomatous germ cell tumour; RTx, radiotherapy; TD, teratoma differentiated.

Pathway/ investigation	A1	A2	A3	B	C	D	E	F	G	H	J	K	L
Outpatient appointment and tumour markers	12	13	5	15	26	10	17	14	23	33	21	7	7
CT scans	1	3	7	4	6	3	2	4	6	7	6	2	3
Chest X-rays	12	9	6	6	8	2	16	11	13	13	11	2	3
Years	5	5	5	5	5	3	10	5	10	10	10	3	3

Figure 19.4 Timing and length of investigations for the 13 follow-up pathways (A1 to L).

recurrence, which (even in standard follow-up) are always detected from patient-reported symptoms, tumour markers and/or radiology results.[7]

Despite some advantages acknowledged in the standard follow-up model of care, from the patient's perspective, the delivery of these services can be challenging. Patients appreciate the value of face-to-face dialogue and interaction with a medical specialist they trust. However, they also understand the pressures on the healthcare system, the problems with brief interactions and the delays in receiving appointments, results and reassurance. Furthermore, travel to a centre with expertise in a rare cancer and the relative lack of flexibility of appointments disrupt patients' daily activities and cause logistical and financial pressures; non-attendance rates are high and appointment rearrangement is frequent.

What are the benefits and challenges of community follow-up?

Patients value community follow-up, especially because of the continuous monitoring of their physical and emotional well-being. PROMs evaluations through QTool promote a comprehensive dialogue with the treatment team which can be accessed in a flexible and straightforward manner. Lengthy travel to the main treatment centre is replaced by a reduced travel time for tests that can be flexibly managed by the patient locally. The patient has control over when investigations are organized, based on their known follow-up schedule. Furthermore, dialogue with the clinical team can be initiated by the patient when reassurance is needed.

This model could also involve some challenges. For instance, there may be a need for better patient information to aid the identification of relevant symptoms and better collaboration between medical centres for timely delivery of investigation results, ensuring continuing timely delivery of results to the patient, as well as continuous design and pragmatic updates to the online system.

How can online assessments of symptoms support community follow-up?

The integration of PROMs into routine clinical care via QTool enhances the patient's clinical assessment.[9] It enables the clinical team to monitor the patient's clinical and psychosocial status. The data are held securely behind the NHS firewall and results are displayed in the patient's electronic record with trends and any concerns. PROMs are assessed in a systematic and standardized manner and their content can be flexibly designed by the clinical team. Based on symptoms relevant in germ cell tumours,[7] the questionnaire asks patients to report their general health, back pain, testicular self-examination, distress levels and causes of distress, such as practical problems (e.g. work, questions about their illness), family (e.g. relationships), emotional problems (e.g. worry, sadness), spiritual concerns (e.g. sense of purpose), and physical problems (e.g. appearance, memory, etc.). It also records the date and location of investigations, supporting the cancer centre to obtain timely results. After a review of data at each assessment, patients receive a letter summarizing their cancer status, or a repeat test or recall to the clinic if concerns arise.

For our patient, all QTool evaluations took place at the required time. Changes in outcomes were readily identified and addressed by the treatment team.

What are patients' opinions of online assessment?

Patients describe QTool as easy to navigate, they appreciate the flexibility of reporting symptoms anywhere, and see the multiple advantages of having a thorough evaluation that will be readily communicated to their treatment team. They feel the online system covers all of their cancer- and treatment-related concerns, which are then readily acted upon by the treatment team without the need for frequent face-to-face appointments. Patients emphasize the importance of timely feedback from the MDT and in future would like the ability to access and monitor their results themselves; this can be achieved via patient portals.

Conclusion and learning points

- There are established evidence-based follow-up pathways for testicular cancer patients, using a traditional model of frequent hospital follow-up visits over 3–10 years.
- Follow-up requires clinical evaluation (including tumour markers, radiological reports and patient reports of symptoms) and holistic assessments of overall well-being and distress.
- Feasible models of risk-stratified and community-supported follow-up care are warranted for the increasing numbers of patients.
- PROMs are straightforward, systematic, cost-effective, and timely in monitoring and addressing patients' symptoms and concerns.
- Patients see self-management advantages in knowing the purpose and timeline of procedures and in having timely reminders and quick results turnaround.
- Patients are satisfied with the new models of follow-up care and can suggest improvements.

References

1 Richards M, Corner J, Maher J. The National Cancer Survivorship Initiative: new and emerging evidence on the ongoing needs of cancer survivors. *Br J Cancer* 2011; 105 (suppl 1): S1–4.

2 Kollmannsberger C, Tandstad T, Bedard PL, *et al.* Patterns of relapse in patients with clinical stage I testicular cancer managed with active surveillance. *J Clin Oncol* 2015; 33: 51–7.

3 Chung P, Daugaard G, Tyldesley S, *et al.* Evaluation of a prognostic model for risk of relapse in stage I seminoma surveillance. *Cancer Med* 2015; 4: 155–60.

4 Dahl AA, Haaland CF, Mykletun A, *et al.* Study of anxiety disorder and depression in long-term survivors of testicular cancer. *J Clin Oncol* 2005; 23: 2389–95.

5 Albers P, Albrecht W, Algaba F, *et al.* EAU guidelines on testicular cancer: 2011 update. *Eur Urol* 2011; 60: 304–19.

6 Cafferty FH, Gabe R, Huddart RA, *et al.* UK management practices in stage I seminoma and the Medical Research Council trial of imaging and schedule in seminoma testis managed with surveillance. *Clin Oncol (R Coll Radiol)* 2012; 24: 25–9.

7 Cunniffe NG, Robson J, Mazhar D, Williams MV. Clinical examination does not assist in the detection of systemic relapse of testicular germ cell tumour. *Clin Oncol (R Coll Radiol)* 2012; 24: 39–42.

8 Harley C, Takeuchi E, Taylor S, *et al.* A mixed methods approach to adapting health-related quality of life measures for use in routine oncology clinical practice. *Qual Life Res* 2012; 21: 389–403.

9 Velikova G, Booth L, Smith AB, *et al.* Measuring quality of life in routine oncology practice improves communication and patient well-being: a randomized controlled trial. *J Clin Oncol* 2004; 22: 714–24.

10 Basch E. Missing patients' symptoms in cancer care delivery – the importance of patient-reported outcomes. *JAMA Oncol* 2016; 2: 433–4.

20 A Young Woman with Advanced Gastric Cancer

Gemma Dart, Alison Young

Case history

A 34-year-old woman with no previous medical history presented with a 6 month history of early satiety, increasing abdominal pain and vomiting. Initial gastroscopy and duodenal biopsies indicated mild reactive gastropathy. She was referred for a diagnostic laparoscopy due to ongoing symptoms and was diagnosed with a stenosing cancer arising at the pylorus and early part of the duodenum. Peritoneal metastases were evident at the point of diagnosis. Biopsies indicated adenocarcinoma. A gastrojejunostomy resolved the pain, vomiting and anorexia caused by the gastric outlet obstruction at presentation.

A referral to medical oncology was requested for consideration of palliative chemotherapy. At the point of diagnosis, the patient and her family requested information on targeted therapies, immunotherapy and intraperitoneal chemotherapies. Following referral there were in-depth discussions about the risks vs benefits of chemotherapy regimens in this setting. The family were keen for further information on potential clinical trials that were not available locally.

The patient's performance status (PS) was 1 at the point of diagnosis, in part due to her poor nutritional state, secondary to previous gastric outlet obstruction and ongoing difficulties with oral nutrition. Her presenting albumin level of 25 g/l continued its downward trend.

There were numerous discussions within the multidisciplinary team (MDT) and with the family regarding the role of parenteral nutrition in this setting. It was felt that a trial of total parenteral nutrition (TPN) prior to consideration of chemotherapy would potentially improve her nutritional state and therefore her PS before cytotoxic treatment. A repeat CT scan indicated a slow pace of change in the disease and clinically she was stable with no new symptoms of concern.

The patient indicated that feeling well and having an improved quality of life (QOL) were the most important immediate aims following diagnosis. She wished to delay palliative chemotherapy until after a family wedding. It was felt that this was a reasonable request and a decision was made to commence TPN in the interim period. Following 2 weeks of TPN a decision was made to proceed with a palliative chemotherapy regimen of oxaliplatin and fluorouracil. She received two cycles of oxaliplatin and bolus fluorouracil and had some improvement in bowel function and pain; however, her overall deterioration continued.

A decision was made not to give further chemotherapy and it was felt that she was unsuitable for review at the trials unit because of her PS 2–3. She was transferred to a hospice for symptom management and she died 6 months following her diagnosis.

What was the goal of cancer treatment for this patient?

What is the evidence base for her treatment options?

How did the patient's comorbidities affect cancer treatment decisions?

How does managing patient expectations change with the complexities of younger patients?

What is the role of TPN in the palliative care setting?

What was the goal of cancer treatment for this patient?

It was clear that treatment options were not curative in nature due to the extent of disease at the point of diagnosis. Consent was taken for palliative chemotherapy with the aim to reduce the size of known metastatic gastric cancer and potentially improve symptom control and prognosis. A holistic approach was taken towards treatment in order to accommodate the patient's wishes. It was also important to review current trial recruitment in the setting of metastatic gastric cancer and consider her eligibility to participate. These considerations were balanced against the optimum time to receive chemotherapy: it was important to ensure she was systemically well enough to tolerate treatment. Repeat imaging prior to decisions being formalized was important to assess the pace of change in the disease alongside the clinical picture.

What is the evidence base for her treatment options?

Careful tumour staging is essential to ensure that patients are appropriately selected for treatment interventions. Standard practice for the management of advanced metastatic gastric cancer is chemotherapy with doublet or triplet platinum plus fluoropyrimidine combinations.[1,2]

- First line treatment:
  - doublet or triplet platinum plus fluoropyrimidine combinations are recommended for fit patients with advanced gastric cancer;[1,3]
  - patients with inoperable locally advanced and/or metastatic (stage IV) disease should be considered for systemic treatment (chemotherapy), which has shown improved survival and QOL compared with best supportive care alone; however, comorbidities, organ function and PS must always be taken into consideration;[1-3]
  - capecitabine is associated with improved overall survival compared with infused fluorouracil in doublet and triplet regimens;[1,4,5]
  - docetaxel, capecitabine and fluorouracil in a 3 weekly regimen was associated with improved overall survival but had significant toxic effects including an increased rate of febrile neutropenia.[1,6]
- Personalized medicine and targeted therapy:
  - trastuzumab is recommended in conjunction with platinum- and fluoropyrimidine-based chemotherapy for patients with human epidermal growth factor receptor 2 (HER2)-positive advanced gastric cancer.[1,7]
- Peritoneal metastases:
  - the use of cytoreductive surgery plus hyperthermic intraperitoneal chemotherapy has been studied in patients with peritoneal metastases, but this approach cannot yet be recommended outside the context of clinical research.[1,8]

- Trials recruiting at the time of patient presentation:
  - the Avelumab in First-Line Maintenance Gastric Cancer (JAVELIN Gastric 100) study is a phase III trial randomizing patients to standard chemotherapy or standard chemotherapy followed by maintenance therapy with avelumab, an anti-programmed death-ligand 1 (PD-L1) antibody;
  - the Study of Pembrolizumab (MK-3475) as First-Line Monotherapy and Combination Therapy for Treatment of Advanced Gastric or Gastroesophageal Junction Adenocarcinoma (MK-3475-062/KEYNOTE-062) is a phase III trial of pembrolizumab as first line monotherapy or combination therapy for the treatment of advanced gastric or gastro-oesophageal junction adenocarcinoma;
  - the Study of Ramucirumab plus Pembrolizumab in Participants with Gastric or GEJ Adenocarcinoma, NSCLC, Transitional Cell Carcinoma of the Urothelium, or Biliary Tract Cancer is a phase I study of ramucirumab plus pembrolizumab in patients with gastric or gastro-oesophageal junction cancer.

Surgery and peritonectomy were also discussed at the point of diagnosis; however, it was felt that due to the extent of disease the response to chemotherapy treatment should be evaluated in the first instance.

How did the patient's comorbidities affect cancer treatment decisions?

Chemotherapy has a number of clinical problems that required assessment and potential intervention. A patient who is unable to maintain an adequate oral intake prior to commencing chemotherapy, due to comorbidities, is less likely to tolerate potential treatment toxicities such as mucositis, nausea and diarrhoea.

Her poor nutritional status, reflected in her body mass index and bloods at diagnosis, was taken into account when discussing potential treatment options. A decision was made to optimize overall nutrition and PS prior to commencing chemotherapy, in order to reduce the risk of toxicity of treatment and potentially improve tolerance of chemotherapy. Owing to concerns surrounding absorption of oral medication and potential bowel obstruction from the extensive peritoneal disease a decision was made within the MDT to proceed with bolus fluorouracil treatment alongside oxaliplatin as opposed to capecitabine treatment. The above was balanced against the patient's young age and prior fitness levels.

How does managing patient expectations change with the complexities of younger patients?

The expectations of this patient and family were apparent from the point of diagnosis. They had researched targeted cancer treatments and their availability in the NHS prior to initial assessment by the oncology team. They were subsequently referred to the phase I trials team to explore these options further. It was important to acknowledge these expectations and be clear that treatment options available for advanced metastatic gastric cancer in the NHS at present are limited and the evidence so far is that they do not significantly alter the poor prognosis of patients presenting with this disease.[1,2]

Although biological therapies and personalized cancer treatment are a rapidly expanding area in medical oncology, it is important to be realistic to patients presenting with an advanced cancer and a poor PS that they may not be eligible for these early-phase trials. Working within the MDT and having a clinical nurse specialist in regular contact with this patient group can potentially improve their cancer journey and psychological acceptance of their illness.

What is the role of TPN in the palliative care setting?

Parenteral nutrition can be used in patients receiving curative treatment for malignancy. Often patients can become malnourished due to the nature of the chemoradiotherapy they are receiving. Oral intake can become difficult and alternative methods of feeding may need to be explored. In the palliative care setting these decisions become much more of a debate. It was clear in this case that parenteral nutrition could not continue indefinitely. The consultations prior to commencement of TPN showed a clear understanding between the clinician and patient that the aim of treatment in this case was to optimize her nutritional state prior to chemotherapy. This decision was taken alongside the nutrition team with input from oncology, pharmacy and the patient.

Although the aims of chemotherapy were palliative in nature, it was important for the patient and her family that she had explored all available options for treatment. The commencement of TPN enabled an improvement in PS prior to treatment; she was therefore able to achieve some personal goals and attend a family wedding that was important for her.

Conclusion and learning points

- Treatment options for advanced metastatic gastric cancer are limited at present. A holistic approach is required to inform the direction of care.

- Patients may attend consultations with expectations of treatment based on their own research, but these need to be balanced with the evidence base available.

- Although it is in an early phase, personalized treatment is becoming more prominent in oncology and in immunotherapy options for gastric cancer and has the potential to transform the management of these difficult tumours.

- TPN can be used to optimize patient PS in the short term; however, it requires careful discussion with all involved to ensure that complications are minimized and that there is a clear aim of treatment and understanding of when it should potentially discontinue.

- Early involvement of the palliative care team and oncology clinical nurse specialist can help to ensure that symptom control and psychological support are considered from an early point in the patient's cancer journey.

References

1 Smyth EC, Verheij M, Allum W, *et al.* Gastric cancer: ESMO clinical practice guidelines. *Ann Oncol* 2016; 27 (suppl 5): v38–49.

2 Glimelius B, Ekström K, Hoffman K, *et al.* Randomized comparison between chemotherapy plus best supportive care with best supportive care in advanced gastric cancer. *Ann Oncol* 1997; 8: 163–8.

3 Wagner AD, Unverzagt S, Grothe W, *et al.* Chemotherapy for advanced gastric cancer. *Cochrane Database Syst Rev* 2010; 3: CD004064.

4 Okines AF, Norman AR, McCloud P, *et al.* Meta-analysis of the REAL-2 and ML17032 trials: evaluating capecitabine-based combination chemotherapy and infused 5-fluorouracil-based combination chemotherapy for the treatment of advanced oesophago-gastric cancer. *Ann Oncol* 2009; 20: 1529–34.

5 Cassidy J, Saltz L, Twelves C, *et al.* Efficacy of capecitabine versus 5-fluorouracil in colorectal and gastric cancers: a meta-analysis of individual data from 6171 patients. *Ann Oncol* 2011; 22: 2604–9.

6 Van Cutsem E, Moiseyenko VM, Tjulandin S, *et al.* Phase III study of docetaxel and cisplatin plus fluorouracil compared with cisplatin and fluorouracil as first line therapy for advanced gastric cancer: a report of the V325 Study Group. *J Clin Oncol* 2006; 24: 4991–7.

7 National Institute for Health and Care Excellence. *Trastuzumab for the treatment of HER2-positive metastatic gastric cancer. Technology appraisal guidance TA208.* London: NICE, 2010.

8 Fujimara T, Yonemura Y, Muroaka K, *et al.* Continuous hyperthermic peritoneal perfusion for the prevention of peritoneal recurrence of gastric cancer: randomised controlled study. *World J Surg* 1994; 18: 150–5.

Further reading

- Allum WH, Blazeby JM, Griffin SM, *et al.* Guidelines for the management of oesophageal and gastric cancer. *Gut* 2011; 60: 1449–72.

- National Institute for Health and Care Excellence. *Gastrointestinal cancers overview.* Available from: https://pathways.nice.org.uk/pathways/gastrointestinal-cancers (accessed 8 June 2017).

21 A Patient with Metastatic Breast Cancer

Alicia-Marie Conway, Elena Takeuchi

Case history

A 48-year-old woman attended a screening mammogram which demonstrated an 8 mm right breast lesion and suspicious axillary lymph nodes. Biopsy of the breast lesion confirmed grade 3 invasive ductal carcinoma, oestrogen receptor (ER) 7, progesterone receptor (PR) 8, human epidermal growth factor receptor 2 (HER2) 1+, with positive axillary nodes. She had a medical history of stage IB malignant melanoma of the upper chest that had been excised 2 years previously. A staging CT revealed a possible solitary bone metastasis in the L5 vertebra, later confirmed on MRI. Biopsy of the L5 lesion confirmed metastatic breast cancer.

During her first medical oncology consultation, her previous mental health issues came to light. She had received treatment for acute psychosis, following a series of family difficulties and a road traffic accident 3 years previously. She had recently been weaned off risperidone and was under psychiatric follow-up. It was clear at this initial consultation that her expectations of treatment were of curative intent and she found discussions of the diagnosis of secondary breast cancer and palliative treatment extremely difficult. The secondary breast care nurses, introduced as part of an integrated palliative care initiative, were able to offer her additional psychological support.

She began first line endocrine therapy with tamoxifen and goserelin, along with denosumab, in view of her low-volume ER-positive metastatic breast cancer. She remained well on endocrine therapy and had no evidence of disease progression in the first 4 months. Given that she had small-volume metastatic disease, a more radical treatment approach was considered. She underwent spinal vertebroplasty followed by surgery to the primary breast tumour. This was followed by postoperative radiotherapy to her right breast.

While undergoing radiotherapy, the patient reported increasing back pain. Restaging investigations unfortunately confirmed rapidly progressive bone disease throughout her spine. Her systemic treatment was changed to first line palliative chemotherapy with capecitabine; she continued bone-directed therapy with denosumab. Her disease remained stable for 6 months; however, she required treatment breaks for palliative radiotherapy and pain control. At the point of progression, her treatment was changed to second line palliative chemotherapy with paclitaxel. A restaging scan after three cycles confirmed further disease progression in her bones.

What was the goal of cancer treatment?

What was the role of the secondary breast care nurse?

What is the evidence for her first line therapy?

What is the evidence for bone-directed therapy?

What is the next step in her metastatic breast cancer management?

What was the goal of cancer treatment?

Metastatic breast cancer is an incurable but treatable disease with average life expectancy of 2–3 years. Some patients with ER-positive, non-visceral metastatic disease may, however, have a better prognosis measurable in terms of several years.

Around 5% of all breast cancer patients are diagnosed with metastatic disease at presentation, and bone metastasis is the most common site. Goals of care in metastatic breast cancer patients are to optimize survival and symptom control and maintain a good quality of life. Treatments should be tailored to the patient's disease and psychosocial needs and priorities, including disease symptoms, body image, employment and family/caring responsibilities, and consideration should be made of how treatment will affect these.[1]

What was the role of the secondary breast care nurse?

At The Christie NHS Foundation Trust, an integrated palliative care approach has been introduced for patients with metastatic breast cancer. Secondary breast care nurses are introduced at the point of diagnosis of metastatic disease to help bridge the gap between active and palliative treatment. This early introduction aims to eliminate any negative perception of palliative care. The team provides holistic support for patients throughout their cancer treatment. Secondary breast care nurses can help guide discussions about treatment and expectations, and identify patients approaching the end of life or in their last year of life.[2]

As this patient had a previous serious psychiatric episode, it was recognized that she may need increased psychological support. Initial discussions from the first discovery of a breast lump were from a curative perspective, but this had changed quickly to palliative treatment in light of her bone metastasis. The patient's previous mental health diagnosis was an important factor when considering management and treatment options. We knew that her previous psychotic episode was triggered by a major stressful life event and that patients with psychotic disorders and schizophrenia are at risk of mental health deterioration during cancer treatment.[3] She had recently been weaned off antipsychotics; if required to restart, antipsychotic medication might have had implications for administration and interaction with chemotherapy agents. It is important that patients with a history of psychiatric disorder are well supported early on and there is close communication between the mental health team and oncologists throughout treatment. It is recommended that early psychiatric assessment can help to deliver high-quality cancer and psychiatric care for such patients.[4]

What is the evidence for her first line therapy?

Endocrine therapy is recommended as first line treatment in patients with ER-positive metastatic breast cancer, particularly in those with low-volume disease or those who do not have significant symptoms arising from their underlying cancer. First line chemotherapy may be more appropriate in patients with a significant disease burden who may have evidence of organ failure, in order to achieve a quick response.[1]

Our patient was premenopausal at the time of her diagnosis. Endocrine therapy with tamoxifen in combination with ovarian suppression (goserelin) was recommended as first line therapy.

Studies have shown significant improvement in progression-free and overall survival when ovarian suppression is combined with tamoxifen, compared with ovarian suppression or tamoxifen alone.[5]

Surgery to the primary tumour in metastatic breast cancer is controversial. There is some evidence to support resection of the primary tumour to improve overall survival and disease control. It is suggested that patients who derive most benefit from surgery to the primary breast tumour are young women with a good performance status who have ER-positive oligometastatic disease.[6] These data, however, are based on retrospective case series; data from prospective randomized trials in support of this suggestion are currently lacking. Current guidelines advise that surgery for primary breast cancer in metastatic breast cancer should not be offered routinely but discussed on a case-by-case basis.[1] It was felt that our patient may derive significant benefit from local disease control by resection of the primary breast tumour.

A patient's response to endocrine therapy is a predictor of endocrine sensitivity. On average, 12 months of progression-free survival may be expected from first line palliative endocrine therapy. Rapidly progressing disease within the first few months of initiating first line endocrine therapy indicates poor endocrine sensitivity as seen in this case. Our patient's disease progressed symptomatically within 6 months of initiating tamoxifen and goserelin; therefore, a change of systemic therapy to chemotherapy was recommended.

What is the evidence for bone-directed therapy?

Denosumab and bisphosphonates help prevent skeletal-related events and bone pain secondary to bone metastasis in metastatic breast cancer.[7] Denosumab was found to be superior to zoledronic acid in terms of delaying and preventing skeletal-related events; denosumab is also easier to administer and does not cause nephrotoxicity.[8] Denosumab is a monoclonal antibody-targeting receptor activator of nuclear factor kappa-B ligand (RANKL); it inhibits osteoclast action and therefore bone resorption. Bisphosphonates are analogues of pyrophosphate and have a direct apoptotic effect on osteoclasts, decreasing bone resorption and increasing bone mineralization through osteoclast inhibition.

Prior to administration of denosumab, vitamin D levels should be checked and replaced to prevent complications with refractory hypocalcaemia. Patients receiving any bone-directed therapy should also have a dental review, and any necessary dental work should be carried out prior to administration to reduce the risk of osteonecrosis of the jaw.

What is the next step in her metastatic breast cancer management?

The patient progressed quickly through two lines of chemotherapy without meaningful disease control. Disease response and duration of disease control with chemotherapy are predictors of survival in metastatic breast cancer. The strongest predictor of response to further lines of chemotherapy is the patient's response to the first two lines of chemotherapy. In addition, successive lines of chemotherapy have decreasing response rates and duration of disease control.[9,10]

Our patient had 6 months of stable disease with capecitabine before her disease progressed in her bones. She had very little benefit from second line chemotherapy with paclitaxel. It was considered unlikely that she would benefit from further chemotherapy. Careful discussions took place with the patient and the focus of her treatment changed from active therapy to symptom control and best supportive care.

Conclusion and learning points

- It is important to confirm the histological diagnosis of metastasis when the primary is uncertain, so that expectations and treatment decisions can be made appropriately.

- An integrated palliative care team approach alongside active treatment can help to support and guide treatment and avoid a crisis in the event of acute change in the clinical situation.

- Endocrine therapy is recommended as first line therapy in ER-positive metastatic breast cancer unless there is evidence of visceral crisis or disease-related symptoms requiring a faster response to treatment.

- Response to previous chemotherapy is the best predictor of response to further lines of chemotherapy in metastatic breast cancer.

- Bone-directed therapy should be prescribed in all patients with bone metastasis to prevent skeletal-related events.

References

1 Cardoso F, Costa A, Norton L, *et al.* ESO-ESMO 2nd international consensus guidelines for advanced breast cancer (ABC2). *Ann Oncol* 2014; 25: 1871–88.

2 Farrell C, Coleby T. An integrated model for breast cancer and palliative care. *Evid Pract* 2016; 15: 7.

3 Irwin KE, Henderson DC, Knight HP, Pirl WF. Cancer care for individuals with schizophrenia. *Cancer* 2014; 120: 323–34.

4 Howard LM, Barley EA, Davies E, *et al.* Cancer diagnosis in people with severe mental illness: practical and ethical issues. *Lancet Oncol* 2010; 11: 797–804.

5 Klijn JG, Blamey RW, Boccardo F, *et al.* Combined tamoxifen and luteinizing hormone-releasing hormone (LHRH) agonist versus LHRH agonist alone in premenopausal advanced breast cancer: a meta-analysis of four randomized trials. *J Clin Oncol* 2001; 19: 343.

6 Ruiterkamp J, Ernst MF. The role of surgery in metastatic breast cancer. *Eur J Cancer* 2011; 47 (suppl 3): S6–22.

7 Van Poznak CH, Temin S, Yee GC, *et al.* American Society of Clinical Oncology executive summary of the clinical practice guideline update on the role of bone-modifying agents in metastatic breast cancer. *J Clin Oncol* 2011; 29: 1221–7.

8 Stopeck AT, Lipton A, Body JJ, *et al.* Denosumab compared with zoledronic acid for the treatment of bone metastases in patients with advanced breast cancer: a randomized, double-blind study. *J Clin Oncol* 2010; 28: 5132–9.

9 Durgresne A, Pivot X, Tournigand C, *et al.* Impact of chemotherapy beyond the first line in patients with metastatic breast cancer. *Breast Cancer Res Treat* 2008; 107: 275–9.

10 Banerji U, Kuciejewska A, Ashley S, *et al.* Factors determining outcome after third line chemotherapy for metastatic breast cancer. *Breast* 2007; 16: 359–66.

22 A Patient with Melanoma, Severe Psychosis on Steroids, and Multiple Other Issues

Hariharan Kuhan, Gail Prout, Paul Nathan

Case history

A 56-year-old woman with a history of *BRAF*-mutant metastatic malignant melanoma excised from her thigh 6 years earlier presented with right-sided sensory disturbance, headache and seizures while under surveillance. An MRI brain scan identified a 3 cm metastasis in the left cerebral hemisphere compressing the corpus callosum, with oedema.

The multidisciplinary team (MDT) felt the metastasis to be amenable to stereotactic radiosurgery (CyberKnife) treatment, in preference to neurosurgery, and she commenced dexamethasone (4 mg twice daily) and anti-seizure medication. Unfortunately, the steroids caused insomnia and paranoid delusions in an acute psychotic episode, requiring lorazepam, antipsychotic drugs and community psychiatric team intervention. Her dexamethasone was carefully reduced to 1 mg daily.

Three months later the patient presented with worsening headaches and blurring of vision; imaging showed disease progression with oedema. Informed consent was obtained to commence the oral systemic serine/threonine-protein kinase B-Raf (BRAF) inhibitor vemurafenib; her dexamethasone dose was increased to 8 mg with increased lorazepam. Risk of toxicities was discussed regularly in clinic consultations and also in telephone conversation with the clinical nurse specialist. Unfortunately, the patient developed grade 3 burns on her hands secondary to photosensitivity caused by the vemurafenib. Vemurafenib was continued for 12 cycles over the course of 1 year. Despite giving excellent intracranial disease control it was discontinued thereafter because of deranged liver function.

Three months later the patient exhibited extracranial disease progression. Recommencement of vemurafenib resulted in a mixed response: shrinkage of some lesions but occurrence of new metastases in the brain. With the continued aid of the clinical nurse specialist, referrals were made to the community Macmillan service, local hospice and eventually a nursing home, as the focus switched from anticancer treatment to best supportive care.

What is the importance of testing *BRAF* mutation status following a diagnosis of malignant melanoma? What is the evidence base for treatment with single-agent BRAF inhibition or combination with a mitogen-activated protein kinase kinase (MEK) inhibitor?

What adverse effects are associated with BRAF inhibitors?

How did the patient's adverse reactions to treatment and comorbidities influence treatment decisions?

What support was made available to the patient and her family by the MDT and community services?

What is the importance of testing *BRAF* mutation status following a diagnosis of malignant melanoma? What is the evidence base for treatment with single–agent BRAF inhibition or combination with a MEK inhibitor?

Approximately 40–60% of cutaneous melanomas carry activating mutations in the *BRAF* gene that lead to constitutive activation of downstream signalling through the mitogen-activated protein kinase (MAPK) pathway. The majority of these mutations result in the substitution of glutamic acid for valine at codon 600 (*BRAF* V600E). Vemurafenib is one of a number of potent inhibitors of mutated *BRAF*. A randomized phase III trial, A Study of Vemurafenib (RO5185426) in Comparison with Dacarbazine in Previously Untreated Patients with Metastatic Melanoma (BRIM-3), showed that vemurafenib improved response and progression-free and overall survival, when compared with dacarbazine chemotherapy in patients with unresectable, previously untreated stage IIIC or stage IV metastatic melanoma with the *BRAF* V600E mutation.[1] Unfortunately, the median time to development of resistance to BRAF inhibitors is 6–8 months. Studies have shown that resistance develops, at least in part, because tumours are able to activate the MAPK/MEK signalling pathway, which allows them to resume growing.[2] Vertical MAPK blockade with combined BRAF and MEK inhibition has greater efficacy. The combination of dabrafenib plus trametinib (a MEK inhibitor) is more active than treatment with a BRAF inhibitor alone.[3-5] Vemurafenib in combination with cobimetinib (a MEK inhibitor) has shown similar benefit,[6] as has the encorafenib/binimetinib combination, and the optimization of combinations is an active area of clinical trials research.

Current NICE guidelines recommend that all patients with non-metastatic but high-risk disease (i.e. those diagnosed with stage IIC or more severe disease using the American Joint Committee on Cancer staging system) should be referred to the specialist skin cancer MDT for review.[7] Patients with stage IIC disease have a 40–70% risk of disease recurrence, mostly 2–4 years after the initial diagnosis. The risk of further metastasis is higher among patients with stage III melanoma. Early *BRAF* mutation testing in high-risk patients allows for rapid initiation of treatment in those who have evidence of disease progression and ensures that the *BRAF* mutation status is known at the time of recurrence for patients originally diagnosed with stage IIC or III disease.[8] Knowledge of *BRAF* mutation status in patients with stage IIC and III disease also facilitates entry into clinical trials where appropriate.

What adverse effects are associated with BRAF inhibitors?

The most common moderate-to-severe adverse events associated with BRAF inhibitor treatment are cutaneous (e.g. rash, keratoacanthoma, cutaneous squamous cell carcinoma and photosensitivity), arthralgia, diarrhoea and fatigue.[9] In BRIM-3,[1] adverse events with the BRAF inhibitor vemurafenib led to dose modification or treatment interruption in 38% of treated patients compared with 16% of patients receiving dacarbazine. There are differences in the side effect profile of different BRAF inhibitors. An extensive international single arm safety study was undertaken which included 3226 patients with advanced melanoma treated with vemurafenib. The most common adverse events of all severity grades associated with vemurafenib were rash (49%), arthralgia (39%), fatigue (34%), photosensitivity (31%), alopecia (26%) and nausea (19%). Forty-six percent of patients experienced grade 3 or 4 adverse events, which were most commonly cutaneous squamous cell carcinoma (12%), rash (5%), liver function abnormalities (5%), arthralgia (3%) and fatigue (3%).[10] The pattern of onset of vemurafenib side effects is predictable: photosensitivity and rash occur usually within days of starting the drug. Arthralgia, diarrhoea, fatigue, alopecia and development of other skin lesions tend to occur over weeks and months. While photosensitivity continues with drug use, other adverse events including rash, skin lesions and arthralgia can regress and be less problematic after the first few months.

The most common dabrafenib-induced adverse events were hyperkeratosis (39%), headache (35%), arthralgia (35%) and pyrexia (32%). Other skin toxicities included keratocanthoma and squamous cell carcinoma (10%), but, unlike with vemurafenib, photosensitivity was extremely rare, indicating this adverse event to be more drug- than class-specific. Grades 3–4 adverse events were uncommon, but pyrexia was identified as a new and potentially significant toxicity occurring in some 5% of treated patients, not commonly seen with vemurafenib.

Interestingly, the combination regimen (BRAF inhibitor plus MEK inhibitors) generates fewer skin toxicities compared with BRAF inhibitor monotherapy. The molecular mechanism is now understood to result from interactions between separate elements of the signal transduction pathway and the two drugs. In the Study Comparing Trametinib and Dabrafenib Combination Therapy to Dabrafenib Monotherapy in Subjects with *BRAF*-mutant Melanoma (COMBI-d) randomized phase III trial, combination therapy was superior to dabrafenib monotherapy.[11] Adverse effects occurred more frequently with combination dabrafenib and trametinib therapy: fever (51%) and chills (30%), fatigue (35%), diarrhoea (24%), hypertension (22%) and vomiting (20%).

How did the patient's adverse reactions to treatment and comorbidities influence treatment decisions?

Unfortunately this patient developed a psychotic disorder, with predominantly manic symptoms, following the use of oral dexamethasone. Although disturbances of mood, cognition, sleep and behaviour as well as frank delirium or even psychosis are possible, the most common adverse effects of short-term corticosteroid therapy are euphoria and hypomania. Corticosteroid-induced symptoms frequently present early in a treatment cycle and typically resolve with dosage reduction or discontinuation of corticosteroids, as we observed in this case.

The patient was evidently sensitive to the psychiatric complications associated with steroid use, including mood and personality disturbance, insomnia and psychosis. In an acute psychotic episode she suffered delusions, including the belief that her husband and family were trying to harm her. Intervention by the crisis resolution and home treatment team was initiated by her oncology team. The clinical nurse specialist had received concerning calls from the patient and her family and, following liaison with the oncology consultant, was swiftly able to make a referral to the community crisis team. There were concerns that the patient was a potential danger to herself and her family. She ultimately required benzodiazepine and an antipsychotic to successfully control these severe side effects of corticosteroids.

Patient education and counselling by the MDT were vital to enable the identification and avoidance of drug toxicities. The patient was advised to avoid direct sun and use sunscreen while on vemurafenib. Unfortunately she experienced photosensitivity burns due to lack of adherence to this advice. Compliance with advice proved difficult in light of the patient's personality but also her family dynamic, which had been strained throughout the various challenges during treatment. Regular clinical nurse specialist input was a necessity to optimize compliance and proved to be an essential 'safety net' for the patient in monitoring for any psychiatric deterioration or social concerns.

The patient was plagued with lymphoedema throughout her treatment, which started following her pelvic lymph node dissection. The lymphoedema was managed with specialist input from the lymphoedema, physiotherapy and occupational therapy teams.

Given her susceptibility to the side effects of systemic treatment an attempt was made to control her intracranial disease by re-treating the solitary area in the brain with stereotactic radiosurgery and spare her drug-induced side effects. Unfortunately, control was short-lived and the patient suffered from disease progression, at which point a decision was made to stop specific anticancer treatment. The patient benefited from early involvement of the palliative care team, which continued in the community. This ensured smoother transition from hospital- to community-based care.

What support was made available to the patient and her family by the MDT and community services?

The clinical nurse specialist acted as a fixed point of contact for the patient throughout diagnosis and treatment. She ensured the patient had access to all necessary community services and was also provided with psychological support and specialist symptom control. Her liaison with the community palliative care team ensured a safe transfer between hospital and community medicine. The role of the clinical nurse specialist was also important in the transition of care goals to best supportive measures, for example when facilitating the patient's request to assist with organizing nursing home placement. There was considerable anxiety at this time, and many interactions with the patient and her family over the phone and in person were essential to aid with the transition.

The many challenges faced over the course of management of her disease had a considerable impact on the patient and her family. The good rapport developed between the oncology team and the patient and her family meant excellent channels of communication were maintained. Although counselling was offered individually to the patient and her family members, when relationships were strained it was not always taken up.

The patient required input from the physiotherapy, occupational therapy and lymphoedema teams because of impaired mobility and risk of falls secondary to her lymphoedema and proximal myopathy. They all had an important role in successfully transitioning the patient from hospital to home in a safe manner but also with ongoing management in the community. The palliative care team was involved at an early stage of her management to help achieve better control of the many effects of the cancer and its treatment. They played a more predominant role as the patient eventually required best supportive care once anticancer treatment was stopped. In the community, the hospice provided holistic care to the patient, addressing symptom control but also acting as an additional support network. There is moderate research evidence to support the role of early specialist palliative care intervention in improvement of symptoms, survival and health-related communication,[12] as was seen in this case.

Conclusion

Patients with advanced cancer often have complex needs requiring multidisciplinary input. Metastatic melanoma patients now have multiple treatment options. This patient's management needs were defined by the interaction between her premorbid psychiatric status and family dynamics, disease-defined symptoms and treatment-related toxicities. All of these issues required active management by a number of professionals, who communicated well with each other and with the patient and her family.

References

1 Chapman P, Hauschild A, Robert C, *et al.* Improved survival with vemurafenib in melanoma with *BRAF* V600E mutation. *N Engl J Med* 2011; 364: 2507–16.

2 Das Thakur M, Salangsang F, Landman A, *et al.* Modelling vemurafenib resistance in melanoma reveals a strategy to forestall drug resistance. *Nature* 2013; 494: 251–6.

3 Flaherty K, Robert C, Hersey P, *et al.* Improved survival with MEK inhibition in *BRAF*-mutated melanoma. *N Engl J Med* 2012; 367: 107–14.

4 Long GV, Stroyakovskiy D, Gogas H, *et al.* Dabrafenib and trametinib versus dabrafenib and placebo for Val600 *BRAF*-mutant melanoma: a multicentre, double-blind, phase 3 randomised controlled trial. *Lancet* 2015; 386: 444–51.

5 Robert C, Karaszewska B, Schachter J, *et al.* Improved overall survival in melanoma with combined dabrafenib and trametinib. *N Engl J Med* 2015; 372: 30–9.

6 Pavlick A, Ribas A, Gonzalez R, *et al.* Extended follow-up results of phase Ib study (BRIM7) of vemurafenib with cobimetinib in *BRAF*-mutant melanoma. *J Clin Oncol* 2015; 33: 9020.

7 National Institute for Health and Clinical Excellence. *Improving outcomes for people with skin tumours including melanoma. Cancer service guideline CSG8.* London: NICE, 2006

8 Gonzalez D, Fearfield L, Nathan P, *et al.* *BRAF* mutation testing algorithm for vemurafenib treatment in melanoma: recommendations from an expert panel. *Br J Dermatol* 2013; 168: 700–7.

9 Welsh SJ, Corrie PG. Management of BRAF and MEK inhibitor toxicities in patients with metastatic melanoma. *Ther Adv Med Oncol* 2015; 7: 122–36.

10 Larkin J, Del Vecchio M, Ascierto P, *et al.* Vemurafenib in patients with *BRAF*(V600) mutated metastatic melanoma: an open-label, multicentre, safety study. *Lancet Oncol* 2014; 15: 436–44.

11 Long G, Stroyakovsky D, Gogas H, *et al.* COMBI-d: a randomized, double-blinded, phase III study comparing the combination of dabrafenib and trametinib to dabrafenib and trametinib placebo as first-line therapy in patients with unresectable or metastatic *BRAF* V600E/K mutation-positive cutaneous melanoma. *J Clin Oncol* 2014; 32 (suppl.): abstract 9011.

12 Salins N, Ramanjulu R, Patra L, *et al.* Integration of early specialist palliative care in cancer care and patient related outcomes: a critical review of evidence. *Indian J Palliat Care* 2016; 22: 252–7.

Index

Note: page numbers in *italics* refer to figures and tables.